WaLKING TWIN CITIES

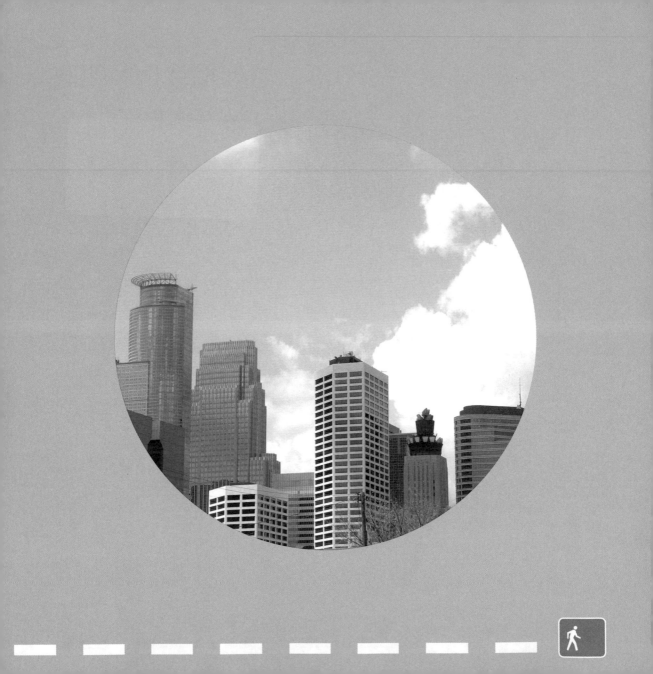

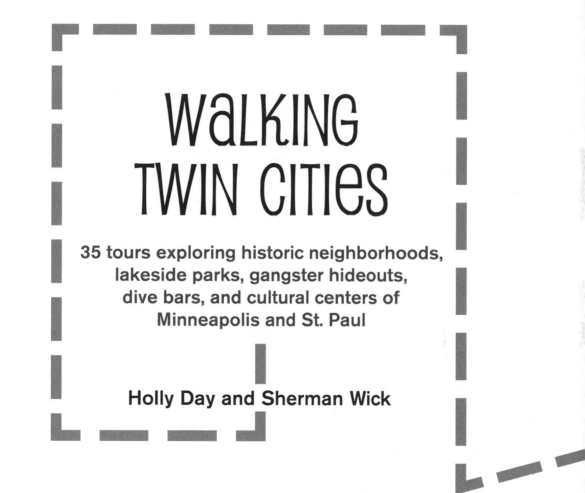

WALKING TWIN CITIES

35 tours exploring historic neighborhoods, lakeside parks, gangster hideouts, dive bars, and cultural centers of Minneapolis and St. Paul

Holly Day and Sherman Wick

WILDERNESS PRESS ... *on the trail since 1967*

Walking Twin Cities: 35 tours exploring historic neighborhoods, lakeside parks, gangster hideouts, dive bars, and cultural centers of Minneapolis and St. Paul

1st EDITION 2009
2nd EDITION 2013

Copyright © 2009, 2013 by Holly Day and Sherman Wick

Cover photos copyright © 2013 by Holly Day and Sherman Wick
Interior photos: Holly Day and Sherman Wick
Maps: Bart Wright, Lohnes + Wright, and Scott McGrew
Book design and layout: Larry B. Van Dyke and Annie Long
Cover design and layout: Larry B. Van Dyke and Scott McGrew

ISBN 978-0-89997-720-1

Manufactured in the United States of America

Published by: **Wilderness Press**
                c/o Keen Communications
                PO Box 43673
                Birmingham, AL 35243
                (800) 443-7227; FAX (205) 326-1012
                info@wildernesspress.com
                www.wildernesspress.com

Visit our website for a complete listing of our books and for ordering information.

Distributed by Publishers Group West

Cover photos: Front, clockwise from bottom center: Minnesota State Capitol; F. Scott Fitzgerald, Rice Park; Broder's Pasta Bar; Minnehaha Falls; downtown St. Paul; Phelps Fountain, Lyndale Park; Lake Phalen. *Back, clockwise from upper right:* James J. Hill House; Gates Ajar, Como Park; Mickey's Dining Car.

Frontispiece: Minneapolis skyline

SAFETY NOTICE: Although Wilderness Press and the authors have made every attempt to ensure that the information in this book is accurate at press time, they are not responsible for any loss, damage, injury, or inconvenience that may occur to anyone while using this book. You are responsible for your own safety and health while following the walking trips described here.

To our grandmothers: Dorothy, Clara, Vera, and Joyce,
for their guidance and inspiration

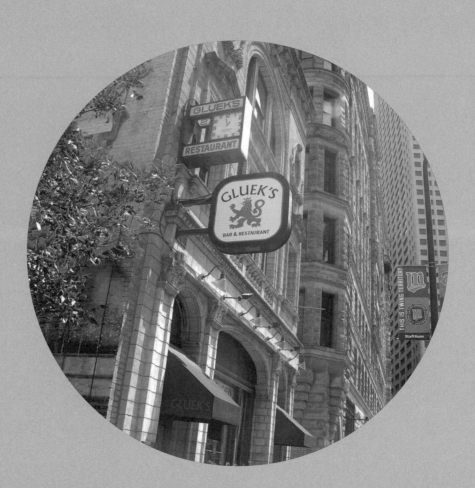

Gluek's Bar & Restaurant

acknowledgments

This edition began on an unusually warm spring day and ended in a likewise unusually warm Indian summer. All of the days that came between only reaffirmed our love/hate relationship with Minnesota's unpredictable weather. The biggest difference between writing this edition and the first was having two kids in school during most of the writing, as opposed to pushing a toddler in a baby stroller for most of the walks. Our thanks go to our two children: Wolfgang and Astrid, who are still both the most open people we know about visiting new places and trying new things. A big thank you goes to our agent, Matt Wagner, and all the people at Wilderness Press for making this book possible.

authors' note

Minnesotans love to talk about the weather—spend any time here, and you'll understand why. A sunny summertime morning can easily turn into a rainy afternoon, and snow can surprise you as late as early May. A good rule of thumb is to check the forecast before heading out, and to make sure that you dress sensibly according to the time of year. Another thing to keep in mind is that as cities evolve, landmarks change. We've tried to mention only landmarks that we're sure will stand the test of time, but you never can account for bad city planning or gentrification.

When navigating Minneapolis, it's especially important to pay attention to the street signs indicating St., Ave., N., S., N.E., S.E., and so on. The city is laid out in a nice, neat grid, but newcomers not used to streets bearing multiple names can get easily lost. St. Paul is a little trickier, due to its poorly plotted street design adapted to a much more difficult, hilly topography. This is why we recommend that visitors and residents alike use the map in the *Hudson's Twin City Street Atlas*; we have included *Hudson's* coordinates for all of the walks in this book.

One new addition to getting around the Twin Cities is the introduction of the ever-expanding Nice Ride bike system, which allows visitors to the Twin Cities to rent bicycles to get from one place to another for a nominal fee without having to resort to driving or taking the bus. This system is a large part of the reason why Minneapolis has been named America's Best Bike City by *Bicycling* magazine. For more information about where to find and check out Nice Ride Bikes, see **niceridemn.org.**

We hope that this book inspires you to investigate the great possibilities the Twin Cities offer. Once again, happy trails!

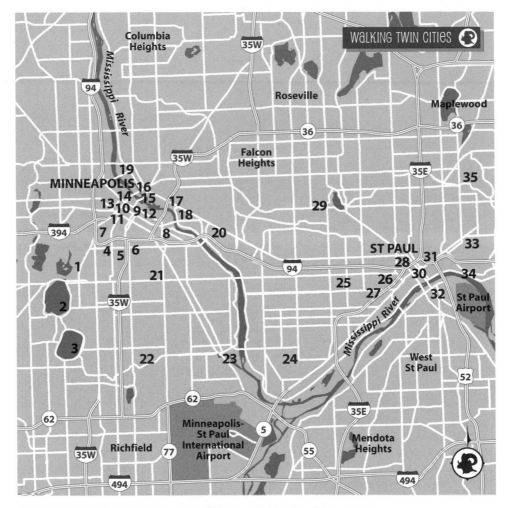

NUMBERS ON THIS LOCATOR MAP CORRESPOND TO WALK NUMBERS.

TABLE OF CONTENTS

INTRODUCTION

Even though they're often lumped together, the Twin Cities are two distinct cities with very different histories. Minneapolis is the Mill City, the City of Lakes, composed mostly of flat prairies. St. Paul is the Capital City, built on rolling hills and high river bluffs.

Culturally, the cities have their differences, too. Minneapolis is home to world-renowned theaters and modern art galleries, while St. Paul is the home of many of the state's institutions, from the seat of government to the seat of the Roman Catholic Archdiocese of St. Paul and Minneapolis. Minneapolis is a newer city, which is reflected in the architecture and overall vibe, while St. Paul's older neighborhoods feature some of the most intact Victorian-era houses in the country. Because of their locations on the west and east sides of the Mississippi River, critics say that Minneapolis is more like a modern West Coast city, while St. Paul is akin to a historic East Coast city.

Both cities are linked by the Mississippi River—the same force that shaped their origins. St. Paul developed earlier, mostly because it was more easily accessible via the river. Thanks to the foresight of the civic-conscious Victorians who succeeded the cities' founders, both cities set aside large tracts of land for public use all along the rivers and lakes. Some of the most beautiful parks were plotted in the early days of the cities.

Even today there are big differences between the cities. For example, St. Paulites, gluttons for punishment, host the annual Winter Carnival during the coldest time of the year. Minneapolitans take the easy way out by celebrating the Aquatennial Festival each summer. Despite having their city festivals at opposite ends of the solstice, Minnesotans love the outdoors. Even with the notoriously fierce winters, Minnesotans statistically spend more time outside than most.

Whether you're interested in art, culture, history, or nature, there's a walk in this book designed for your interests. We hope that it serves not only as a guidebook for (re)discovering the Twin Cities but also as a springboard for additional explorations.

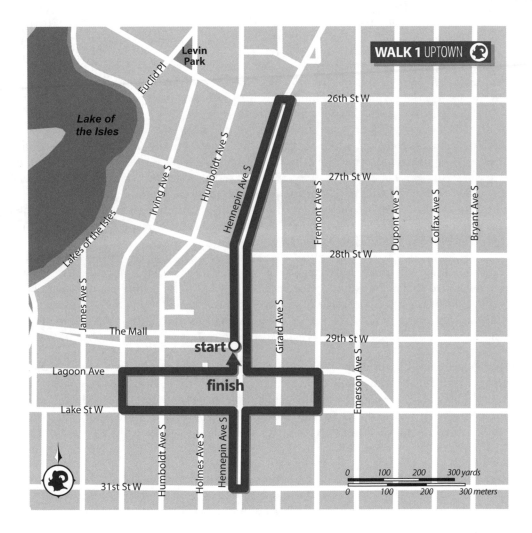

1 UPTOWN: COOL PLACE FOR FUN IN THE HOT SUMMER SUN

BOUNDARIES: **31st St. W., Irving Ave. S., 26th St. W., Fremont Ave. S.**
HUDSON'S TWIN CITY STREET ATLAS COORDINATES: **Map 394, 1D**
DISTANCE: **Approx. 1½ miles**
DIFFICULTY: **Easy**
PARKING: **Free parking on The Mall**
PUBLIC TRANSIT: **Numerous bus lines to Uptown Station (Located at Hennepin Ave. S. and the end of The Mall)**

Uptown is the Twin Cities' place for fun—especially during summertime. It's not officially recognized as a neighborhood by the City of Minneapolis, and it's actually composed of sections of the Calhoun, East Calhoun, East Isles, and Lowry East neighborhoods. It became a de facto second downtown after Calhoun Square opened in 1983, combining extant buildings and new constructions to create an urban shopping center. With its almost endless array of entertainment options—including bars, coffee shops, restaurants, music clubs, comedy clubs, movie theaters, art galleries, shopping, and tattoo parlors—the area attracts hip, young crowds. The proximity to Lake Calhoun and Lake of the Isles only heightens the cachet of the area during warm weather, when, after a day at the beach, locals enjoy the neighborhood amenities. Put all these together and it makes for a fun and often playfully raucous neighborhood—and a great place for a walk.

● Begin at the west corner of Uptown Station (bus stop) and turn left heading north on Hennepin Ave. S. As you follow the gradual slope downhill, notice the funky grandeur of this stretch of Uptown, an often incongruent combination of architectural styles where beautifully restored storefronts sit uneasily beside cookie-cutter strip mall buildings. In recent years, more national chain businesses have appeared.

● Turn right on 26th St. W. and immediately turn right again going south on Hennepin Ave. S. Continue south on Hennepin as the avenue cuts through the grid at Girard Ave. S., passing the Mount Royal Apartments. On the left is Saint Sabrina's, the professional tattooing and ear- and body-piercing parlor. After opening in 1993, the parlor moved to the new location in 2006 and slightly de-emphasized the purgatory and hell themes. Free coffee, tea, and movies are offered to customers in a comfortable and relaxed atmosphere.

- Cross 28th St. W. On the left, as you continue on the east side of the street, the Tibet Store sells the best from the spiritual homeland of the Dalai Lama. The store stocks reasonably priced clothing, as well as jewelry and Tibetan Buddhist books. Just ahead down the hill is the Williams Uptown Pub & Peanut Bar. This popular hangout serves 300 different bottled brews and 70 different draft beers with good bar food upstairs. Free popcorn, peanuts, games, and darts are available in the basement. Kitty-corner on Lagoon Ave. is the marquee of the recently renovated Moderne-style Landmark's Uptown Theatre, a gateway to the business district since 1939.

- Turn left on Lagoon Ave. At the corner of Girard Ave. S. is the Uptown's sister theater—Landmark Theatres' Lagoon Cinema, with five screens specializing in art house, indie, and foreign films.

- Turn right on Fremont Ave. S. To the left is the oddball color scheme of the New Traditionalist–style Uptown City Apartments.

- Turn right on Lake St. W. Kitty-corner is Tum Rup Thai, a perennially award-winning restaurant with all the Thai standards such as spring rolls, pad Thai, and curries, plus numerous fresh seafood and vegetarian items. Adventurous lovers of

UPTOWN art Fair: art & SUN

Uptown is the summer-fun place for the Twin Cities, and the annual Uptown Art Fair is the pinnacle of seasonal merriment. Locals and visitors from around the world enjoy one of the Midwest's premier fine-art festivals, usually scheduled for the first weekend in August—one of the few times when warm weather is almost guaranteed. With 450 artists juried and evaluated by professionals, the quality of the exhibitors' art is as excellent as it is diverse, and includes something for almost anyone. There are incredible people-watching opportunity as more than 300,000 visitors descend for the three-day weekend event. The first Uptown Art Fair was held in 1963, and it attracted a small enthusiastic crowd. Over time, the event grew—too large by the early 1990s when more than 600 exhibitors displayed their wares; since then it has become more selective and competitive. It remains a favorite event for those browsing for art or simply enjoying summer in the Twin Cities.

seafood need to try the Bangkok Sea Breeze, a mountain of fresh shrimp, scallops, squid, and mussels in a spicy sauce—enormous enough to feed two, and even better with a beer or a mixed drink.

- Cross Girard Ave. S. and go straight to get to Stella's Fish Café & Prestige Oyster Bar. There you'll get fresh seafood and plenty of alcohol in this lovely renovated restaurant with rooftop dining and lots of hip, young things in the summer.

- Turn left on Hennepin Ave. S. where Calhoun Square is located. Uptown became an essential shopping destination after this retail center opened. Unfortunately, in recent years business has waned, and it has gone through a succession of ownership groups which have tried to reinvent the center.

- Turn right on 31st St. W. and right again on Hennepin Ave. S. Just past the stunning and unusual Spanish Churrigueresque Revival façade of the now-closed Suburban World Theatre (1927) is the former site of the Uptown Bar and Café, once a popular performance space for local and national bands and now a big-box store.

- Turn left on Lake St. W. after passing a half block of invading national chains. On the right is Mesa Pizza, a satellite of the popular pizza place in Dinkytown, selling cheap pizza by the slice until the late-night hours.

- Turn right on Irving Ave. S. On the northwest corner of Lake St. is Barbette—fine dining for cool folks.

- Turn right on Lagoon Ave.

- Turn left on Hennepin Ave. S. and finish the walk at Uptown Station.

POINTS OF INTEREST

Saint Sabrina's saintsabrinas.com, 2645 Hennepin Ave. S., Minneapolis, MN 55408, 612-874-7360

Tibet Store tibetstorempls.com, 2835 Hennepin Ave. S., Minneapolis, MN 55408, 612-872-8800

Williams Uptown Pub & Peanut Bar williamsminneapolis.com, 2911 Hennepin Ave. S., Minneapolis, MN 55408, 612-823-6271

Uptown Theatre landmarktheatres.com/market/minneapolis/uptowntheatre.htm, 2906 Hennepin Ave. S., Minneapolis, MN 55408, 612-825-6006

Lagoon Cinema landmarktheatres.com/market/minneapolis/lagooncinema.htm, 1320 Lagoon Ave., Minneapolis, MN 55408, 612-825-6006

Tum Rup Thai tumrupthai.com, 1221 Lake St. W., Minneapolis, MN 55408, 612-824-1378

Stella's Fish Café & Prestige Oyster Bar stellasfishcafe.com, 1400 Lake St. W., Minneapolis, MN 55408, 612-824-8862

Calhoun Square calhounsquare.com, 3001 Hennepin Ave. S., Minneapolis, MN 55408, 612-824-1240

Mesa Pizza Uptown mesapizzamn.com, 1440 Lake St. W., Minneapolis, MN 55408, 612-206-3206

Barbette barbette.com, 1600 Lake St. W., Minneapolis, MN 55408, 612-827-5710

route summary

1. Begin at the west corner of Uptown Station (bus stop) and turn left heading north on Hennepin Ave. S.
2. Turn right on 26th St. W. and immediately turn right again on Hennepin Ave. S.
3. Continue heading south on Hennepin Ave. S., crossing 28th St. W.
4. Turn left on Lagoon Ave.
5. Go right on Fremont Ave. S.
6. Turn right on Lake St. W.
7. Turn left on Hennepin Ave. S. where Calhoun Square is located.
8. Turn right on 31st St. W. and right again on Hennepin Ave. S.
9. Turn left on Lake St. W. after passing a half block of national chains.
10. Turn right on Irving Ave. S.
11. Turn right on Lagoon Ave.
12. Turn left on Hennepin Ave. S. and finish the walk at Uptown Station.

Fresh seafood on the rooftop at Stella's

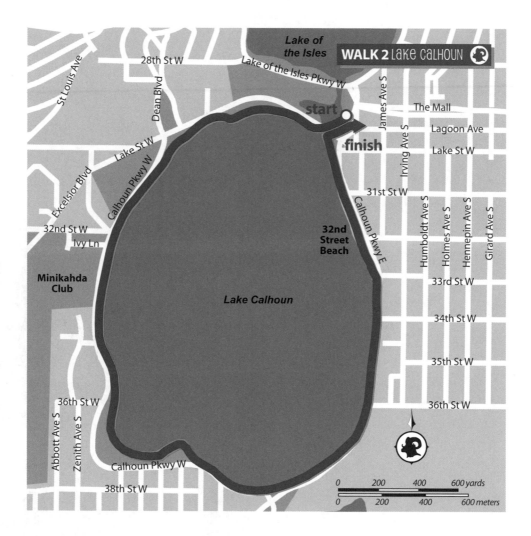

WALK 2 Lake Calhoun

Lake of the Isles

28th St W

Lake of the Isles Pkwy W

St Louis Ave

Dean Blvd

start

finish

James Ave S

The Mall

Lagoon Ave

Irving Ave S

Lake St W

Lake St W

Calhoun Pkwy W

Excelsior Blvd

31st St W

32nd St W

Ivy Ln

Calhoun Pkwy W

Humboldt Ave S

Holmes Ave S

Hennepin Ave S

Girard Ave S

32nd Street Beach

Calhoun Pkwy E

33rd St W

Minikahda Club

Lake Calhoun

34th St W

35th St W

36th St W

36th St W

Abbott Ave S

Zenith Ave S

Calhoun Pkwy W

38th St W

0   200   400   600 yards

0   200   400   600 meters

2 Lake Calhoun: Biggest Pearl in the Chain of Lakes

BOUNDARIES: Calhoun Pkwy. E., Lake St. W., Lagoon Ave., Irving Ave., Calhoun Pkwy. W.
HUDSON'S TWIN CITY STREET ATLAS **COORDINATES:** Map 393, 5D; Map 420, 5A; Map 394, 1D
DISTANCE: Approx. 3¼ miles
DIFFICULTY: Easy but long
PARKING: Free parking on The Mall, located at Mall and Knox Ave. S.
PUBLIC TRANSIT: Bus lines 23, 114, and 115

Lake Calhoun is the largest lake in Minneapolis's popular Chain of Lakes system, which includes Lake Harriet, Brownie Lake, Lake of the Isles, and Cedar Lake. Calhoun is also a part of the Grand Rounds Scenic Byway, a 50 mile route that connects many of Minneapolis's parks and lakes. Theoretically, with only a few tiny gaps in the circuit, you can travel from park to park by foot or bicycle via the Grand Rounds without ever having to get in a car. All around Lake Calhoun are sandy, well-maintained beaches, perfect for swimming or just lying out in the sun—or, if you'd prefer, you can take a break from walking and rent a canoe or paddleboat instead.

- Start across the street from the corner of Mall and Knox Ave. S. Go straight, briefly heading west before the path curves south, toward the water and to your left.

- Take your first left to walk along Lake Calhoun. Off to your right is the path leading to Lake of the Isles, which is another great bird-watching and hiking area.

- At the fork, keep to the right to continue following the lake on the walking path. To your left is a little marsh where you might see baby wood ducks and mallards in late spring and early summer, while to the right is the full arc of the lake. During hot and dry summers, the water level can get low enough so that the waterway becomes choked with duckweed and water lilies; when the season is wet and rainy, many of these paths become completely submerged.

- Go under the Lake Street Bridge and keep going straight. Follow the path up the hill.

- At the canoe rental and boat launch, turn left just before the boat launch and go up the hill toward the street.

- Turn left to follow Lake St. W. to go over the bridge that you just walked under. Stay on the left side of the path marked with the pedestrian sign or you'll get clobbered by a passing bicyclist.

- Follow the pedestrian path down the hill and continue on the path to follow the lake-shore. All summer long, this is the place to watch sailboats and other human- and wind-powered crafts on the lake. In the wintertime, a few hardy individuals head out onto the frozen surface of the lake to go ice sailing, which is a lot like windsurfing only on ice.

- Follow the curve of the lake until the shoreline gets sandy. You can leave the concrete path to walk along the beach, as both paths lead in the same direction. The sandy path opens up into Lake Calhoun North Beach, a popular swimming beach complete with lifeguard. If you brought a towel along, this is a great place for a dip—or just roll your pants up for a knee-deep wade.

- Follow the path past the beach and keep going straight. To the right is a children's playground, and if you have any kids with you, this is a great diversion. Keep going straight to follow the lakeshore. To the left, the sandy shore turns into boulders, only recently installed by the city to protect the shoreline from further erosion.

- Keep following the shoreline. After a while, the right side of the street becomes lined with tree-covered bluffs, and for the next couple of blocks every house on your right is a grand mansion—new or old. At the end of the block are the sprawling grounds of the Bakken: A Library and Museum of Electricity in Life. The gigantic yellow brick-and-stone fortress was originally designed by entrepreneur William Goodfellow in the 1930s to impress a woman who called him cheap. The museum has an amazing collection of antique electrical instruments used for musical and scientific purposes. You can easily access the Bakken from here—the first fork in the path (at 36th St. W.) heads off to the right toward the museum.

- Go straight past the fork to continue along the lakeshore. To your right is a large picnic area, with tables and a sand volleyball court. In the summer, the grounds here are packed with park-goers enjoying the hot sun and cool breezes coming off the water.

- Go straight at the next fork to continue following the lakeshore. Just past the parking lot is Thomas Beach, another popular swimming beach.

- Cross the path driveway to continue on. At the side of the path is a pump-operated drinking fountain with a dog bowl, from which four-footed hikers can drink.

  From here, you get a great view of downtown Minneapolis on the far side of the lake, and to the side of the downtown skyline you can see the distinctive dome of St. Mary's Greek Orthodox Church. Up ahead and to your left, you'll see a little wooden dock. If you like to fish, come early or be prepared to share the dock with other avid fishermen. To your right, just past the fishing dock, is the Lake Calhoun archery range, and just past it is historic Lakewood Memorial Cemetery. The 125-year-old cemetery is absolutely huge; it's open to the public seven days a week, year-round.

- Keep following the path. On your right, keep an eye out for the boulder that marks the first dwelling in what would become Minneapolis. This marker commemorates the spot where Samuel W. and Gideon Pond, who came to Minnesota to convert American Indians to Christianity, built their mission in 1834. The gold-domed St. Mary's Greek Orthodox Church up the hill at 3450 Irving Ave. S. was built virtually on top of the Ponds' original mission in 1957.

- Keep going straight. Up the first set of stairs and to the right is the Minnesota Zen Meditation Center. Open to the public, it offers classes on meditation as well as quiet garden spots perfect for individual practice. You'll also find Lake Calhoun's newest swimming beach here, the 32nd Street Beach.

- Continue due north, following the curve of the lake, until you reach the white, red-roofed park pavilion. At the pavilion, you can get good, reasonably priced seafood at The Tin Fish. There's no indoor dining here, but plenty of picnic tables look right out over the lake. You can also rent a canoe or paddleboat, or go for a gondola ride from the pavilion.

- From the pavilion, go straight past the canoe/paddleboat rentals and onto the walking path to follow the shoreline.

- Go straight in a northerly direction on the pedestrian path and under the Lake Street Bridge.

- Follow the path past the marshland and take your first right.

- Go straight to the street crossing of Mall and Knox Ave. S.—and you're back where you started.

POINTS OF INTEREST

Lake Calhoun North Beach tinyurl.com/calhounnorth, 2710 Lake St. W., Minneapolis, MN 55417, 612-230-6400

The Bakken: A Library and Museum of Electricity in Life thebakken.org, 3537 Zenith Ave. S., Minneapolis, MN 55416, 612-926-3878

Thomas Beach tinyurl.com/thomasbeach, Thomas Ave. S and Calhoun Pkwy. W., Minneapolis, MN 55417, 612-230-6400

Lakewood Memorial Cemetery lakewoodcemetery.com, 3600 Hennepin Ave., Minneapolis, MN 55408, 612-822-2171

St. Mary's Greek Orthodox Church stmarysgoc.org, 3450 Irving Ave. S., Minneapolis, MN 55408, 612-825-2247

Minnesota Zen Meditation Center mnzencenter.org, 3343 Calhoun Pkwy. E., Minneapolis, MN 55408, 612-822-5313

32nd Street Beach tinyurl.com/32ndbeach, 3200 Calhoun Pkwy. E., Minneapolis, MN 55417, 612-230-6400

The Tin Fish thetinfish.net, 3000 Calhoun Pkwy. E., Minneapolis, MN 55408, 612-823-5840

route summary

1. Start across the street from the corner of The Mall and Knox Ave. S. Go straight down the path heading toward the water and to your left.

2. Take your first left to walk along Lake Calhoun.

3. At the fork, keep to the right to continue following the lake.

4. Go under the Lake Street Bridge and keep going straight. Follow the path up the hill.

5. Turn left just before you pass the boat launch, and go up the hill toward the street.

6. Turn left to follow Lake St. and stay on the left side of the path.

7. Follow the pedestrian path down the hill and along the curve of the lake.

8. Go past Lake Calhoun North Beach, Thomas Beach, and 32nd Street Beach, and go to the pavilion.

9. From the pavilion, go straight past the canoe/paddleboat rentals and onto the walking path to follow the shoreline.

10. Continue straight on the pedestrian path to go under the Lake Street Bridge.

11. Follow the path past the marshland and take your first right.

12. Go straight to the street crossing of The Mall and Knox Ave. S., the starting point.

Boats on Lake Calhoun

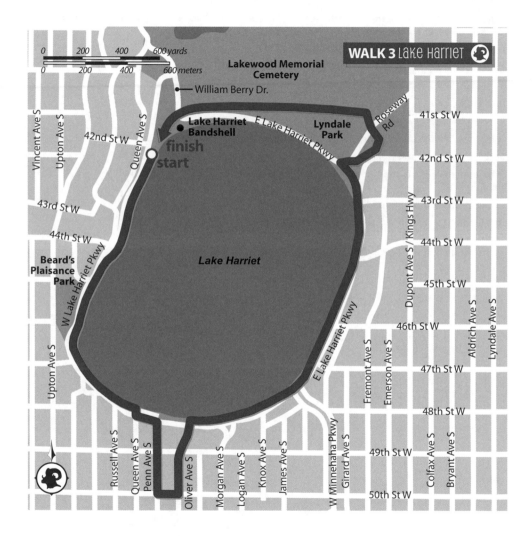

0   200   400   600 yards
0   200   400   600 meters

Lakewood Memorial
Cemetery

William Berry Dr.

Lake Harriet
Bandshell

E Lake Harriet Pkwy

Lyndale
Park

Roseway Rd

Vincent Ave S

Upton Ave S

42nd St W

Queen Ave S

finish
start

41st St W

42nd St W

43rd St W

43rd St W

44th St W

44th St W

Beard's
Plaisance
Park

Lake Harriet

45th St W

W Lake Harriet Pkwy

E Lake Harriet Pkwy

Dupont Ave S / Kings Hwy

46th St W

Upton Ave S

47th St W

Aldrich Ave S

Lyndale Ave S

Fremont Ave S

Emerson Ave S

48th St W

Russell Ave S

Queen Ave S

Penn Ave S

Oliver Ave S

Morgan Ave S

Logan Ave S

Knox Ave S

James Ave S

W Minnehaha Pkwy

Girard Ave S

49th St W

Colfax Ave S

Bryant Ave S

50th St W

3 Lake Harriet: WILDLIFE IN THE HEART OF THE CITY

BOUNDARIES: 50th St. W., W. Lake Harriet Pkwy., William Berry Dr., Kings Hwy., E. Lake Harriet Pkwy.

HUDSON'S TWIN CITY STREET ATLAS COORDINATES: **Map 420, 5A and 5B; Map 421, 1A and 1B**

DISTANCE: **Approx. 3½ miles**

DIFFICULTY: **Moderate**

PARKING: **Free parking on Lake Harriet Pkwy. and nearby side streets**

PUBLIC TRANSIT: **Bus line 4**

You may have noticed that a few sites in the Twin Cities bear the name Harriet. As a general rule, the Harriet sites in St. Paul are named after Harriet Bishop, who was the first school-teacher in St. Paul, while the Harriet sites in Minneapolis are named after Harriet Lovejoy, the wife of Colonel Henry Leavenworth. According to legend, Leavenworth missed his wife very much while he was stationed at Fort Snelling, so he named just about anything beautiful that he came across after her.

Today, Lake Harriet is still one of the loveliest lakes in the region, attracting throngs of park-goers all year long. Along the banks of the lake are hiking and biking trails, benches for bird-watching, places to eat, and, of course, the historic Lake Harriet Bandshell, which features live music every evening from spring to fall. Nearby are the Lyndale Park Rose Gardens, historic Memorial Cemetery, Lyndale Park Peace Garden, Como–Harriet Streetcar Line, and Roberts Bird Sanctuary.

● Start at the LAKE HARRIET park sign, just south of the corner of 42nd St. W. and W. Lake Harriet Pkwy.

● Facing the lake, make a right to walk along the lakeshore. In early spring you'll see flocks of loons migrating north; mallards, seagulls, wood ducks, and Canada geese are present all spring and summer long. All along the lake numerous benches face the water, so if you want to stop and simply take in everything, there are lots of comfortable places to sit. To your right is the Twin Cities historic streetcar line. If you enjoy fishing, try out one of the many spots for shore fishing along the banks here. The first set of steps you pass leads up to Beard's Plaisance Park, with public tennis courts, a picnic area, and a hilltop pavilion that can be reserved for special occasions.

- Keep following the path around the lake. Just past the long fishing pier to your left, you'll pass a group of marshy islands and a little scenic overlook. This is a great spot to see ducks and geese as well as their offspring.

- Cross the little wooden bridge and keep following the curve of the shoreline. You can see the scope of the Lake Harriet Bandshell and, in the summer, dozens of sailboats across the lake from here.

- Take the first tall set of steps to your right and go all the way to the top to Queen Ave. S. and Lake Harriet Pkwy.

- Cross the street and turn left to follow Lake Harriet Pkwy.

- At Penn Ave. S., turn right. This takes you through the modern, upscale Lynnhurst neighborhood, where McMansions are constantly springing up.

- Cross 49th St. W. and keep going straight. At the bottom of the hill is a little neighborhood business district, with the excellent Italian restaurants Broder's Pasta Bar and Broder's Cucina Italiana. Broder's Pasta Bar is an intimate and elegant Italian restaurant that opens only for dinner, with items such as crab lasagna and stuffed mussels on its menu. Across the street, the Cucina carries the same quality of food as the Pasta Bar but serves it in a more relaxed, café-style setting.

- Turn left at 50th St. W.

- Turn left at Oliver Ave S., heading north.

- Cross the street at Lake Harriet Pkwy. and take the steps all the way down to the walking path below. You can see the Lake Harriet Pavilion and the downtown Minneapolis skyline far across on the other side of the lake.

- Turn right to follow the walking path around the lake. To your right are some of the most magnificent mansions along this walk.

At the green water pump is Lake Harriet Southeast Beach, a small swimming beach.

● Continue on the path around the lakeshore. When you pass the boat racks on your left, take the right fork and cross E. Lake Harriet Pkwy. Make an immediate right again to cross Roseway Rd.

● Cut through the grass down the hill to get to the little path at the bottom. Take the path through the gate and go straight.

You are now inside the Lyndale Park Rose Garden, the second-oldest public rose garden in the United States. The garden was designed by Theodore Wirth—also the designer of the country's oldest public rose garden in Connecticut—who served as parks superintendent for Minneapolis 1906–1938 and designed most of the city's fabulous parks.

● Head north through the rose garden and around the Italian Heffelfinger Fountain. Turn left to walk alongside the Lyndale Park Perennial and Annual Display Garden, built in 1963 when the Phelps Fountain (the one with the turtles, located straight ahead) was moved here from Gateway Park in downtown Minneapolis. The garden contains hundreds of exotic and native plants, all clearly identified.

● Follow the gravel path to the right and turn left at the sidewalk to cross Roseway Rd. To your right is the Lyndale Park Peace (Rock) Garden, containing a wide variety of pine trees from all over the world, as well as willows, grasses, and thousands of flower varieties.

Phelps Fountain in Lyndale Park

- Follow the sidewalk to the parking lot. Go straight to pass through the little wooden structure and enter the Thomas Sadler Roberts Bird Sanctuary, named after the notable ornithologist whose 1919 book, *A Review of the Ornithology of Minnesota,* is still one of the best-selling Minnesota-themed bird books of all time.

- Turn right to go onto the plank pathway and follow it through the sanctuary. While you might not be able to see many birds inside, you'll certainly hear hundreds of them all around you.

- Take a left at the end of the plastic boardwalk. To your left are dense reed- and cattail-filled wetlands, home to orioles, red-winged blackbirds, and other songbirds; to your right is a swampy marsh where you can usually spot waterfowl families.

- Go straight to the second plastic boardwalk and turn right. This takes you directly through the marsh, where you can get a closer look at some of the waterbirds that live here. Be careful through the last part of the boardwalk, as flooding sometimes causes it to dip underwater as you're walking over it.

- Turn left at the end of the boardwalk. To your left is another waterfowl nesting site, as well as the back end of Lakewood Memorial Cemetery. The fallen trees in the dense forest nearby have been intentionally left to naturally compost. In the hot, sweaty days of late summer, you can see some spectacular bright orange and yellow bracket mushrooms on many of the dead logs.

- Go straight past the fork to follow the Lakewood Memorial Cemetery fence. Go through the gate and up the stairs to the street.

- Cross the street to the parking lot. Continue heading west, straight through the lot, and cut across the bicycle path (watch for zooming bicyclists) until you get to the pedestrian path.

- Turn left slightly on the path. This takes you by the Lake Harriet Bandshell, officially the fifth music pavilion to be built on this site since the original was erected in 1888. The restrooms to your right were built in 1891 but fortunately feature completely modern facilities inside. Picnic tables are up the hill from here to your right.

- Follow the sidewalk toward the lake. The smaller building by the band shell has more restrooms inside, as well as a small walk-up window where you can buy hot dogs, coffee, sodas, and ice cream. There's no indoor dining, but many picnic tables nearby look out onto the water.

- Follow the path to the right and go straight. Up to the right at the top of the hill is the station for the Como–Harriet Streetcar Line, which takes passengers down the last remaining original tracks of the famed Twin Cities streetcar line to Lakewood Memorial Cemetery and back. (Note that the streetcar line operates only May–October on select days; check the website below for its schedule.) Straight ahead of you is the LAKE HARRIET sign, the starting point.

POINTS OF INTEREST

Beard's Plaisance Park tinyurl.com/beardsplaisance, 45th St. W. and Upton Ave. S., Minneapolis, MN 55419, 612-230-6400

Broder's Pasta Bar broders.com, 5000 Penn Ave. S., Minneapolis, MN 55419, 612-925-9202

Broder's Cucina Italiana broders.com, 2308 50th St. W., Minneapolis, MN 55419, 612-925-3113

Lake Harriet Southeast Beach tinyurl.com/SEbeach, 4740 Lake Harriet Pkwy. E., Minneapolis, MN 55417, 612-230-6400

Lyndale Park tinyurl.com/lyndalepark, 4124 Roseway Rd., Minneapolis, MN 55409, 612-230-6400

Lakewood Memorial Cemetery lakewoodcemetery.com, 3600 Hennepin Ave., Minneapolis, MN 55408, 612-822-2171

Lake Harriet Bandshell tinyurl.com/harrietlake, 43rd St. W. and W. Lake Harriet Pkwy., Minneapolis, MN 55409, 612-230-6400

Como–Harriet Streetcar Line trolleyride.org, 2330 42nd St. W., Minneapolis, MN 55410, 651-228-0263

route summary

1. Start at the LAKE HARRIET sign, just south of the corner of 42nd St. W. and W. Lake Harriet Pkwy.
2. Facing the lake, make a right to walk along the lakeshore.
3. Follow the lakeshore past the fishing pier and over the wooden bridge until you reach the first set of steps to your right going up to street level.
4. Go up the stairs and cross the street.
5. Turn left to follow Lake Harriet Pkwy.
6. Turn right at Penn Ave. S. and go straight.
7. Turn left at 50th St. W. and go straight.
8. Turn left at Oliver Ave. S. and go straight.
9. Cross the street at 49th St. W. and go straight.
10. Cross the street at Lake Harriet Pkwy. and take the steps all the way down to the walking path below.
11. Turn right onto the walking path and follow the path around the lake.
12. Just past the boat racks on your left, take the right fork of the path.
13. Cross E. Lake Harriet Pkwy. and make an immediate right again to cross Roseway Rd.
14. Cut through the grass down the hill to get to the path at the bottom. Take the path through the gate and go straight into the Lyndale Park Rose Garden.
15. Go straight through the rose garden and around the Heffelfinger Fountain.
16. Turn left to walk alongside the Lyndale Park Perennial and Annual Display Garden.
17. Follow the gravel path to the right and turn left at the sidewalk to cross Roseway Rd.
18. Follow the sidewalk to the parking lot and go straight through the lot to the wooden structure; enter the Thomas Sadler Roberts Bird Sanctuary.
19. Turn right to go onto the plank pathway.
20. At the end of the plastic boardwalk, take a left and go straight.
21. Go straight to the second plastic boardwalk and turn right.
22. Turn left at the end of the boardwalk and go straight.
23. Go straight past the fork to follow the Lakewood Memorial Cemetery fence.
24. Go through the gate and up the stairs to the street.
25. Go straight across the street to the parking lot.
26. Go through the lot, past the bicycle path, and onto the pedestrian path.
27. Follow the sidewalk toward the lake.
28. Follow the path to the right and go straight. Straight ahead of you is the LAKE HARRIET sign, the starting point.

Grab some takeout at Broder's Cucina Italiana.

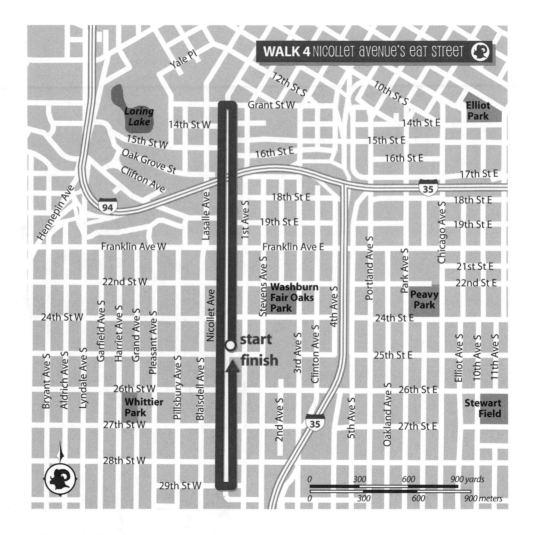

Yale Pl

12th St S

10th St S

Grant St W

14th St W

Loring Lake

Elliot Park

14th St E

15th St W

15th St E

Oak Grove St

16th St E

16th St E

Clifton Ave

17th St E

Hennepin Ave

94

18th St E

18th St E

Lasalle Ave

1st Ave S

19th St E

19th St E

Franklin Ave W

Franklin Ave E

22nd St W

Stevens Ave S

Washburn Fair Oaks Park

Portland Ave S

Park Ave S

Chicago Ave S

21st St E

22nd St E

Peavy Park

24th St W

Garfield Ave S

Harriet Ave S

Grand Ave S

Pleasant Ave S

Nicollet Ave

24th St E

Bryant Ave S

Aldrich Ave S

Lyndale Ave S

Pillsbury Ave S

Blaisdell Ave S

start finish

3rd Ave S

Clinton Ave S

4th Ave S

25th St E

Elliot Ave S

10th Ave S

11th Ave S

26th St W

Whittier Park

2nd Ave S

5th Ave S

Oakland Ave S

26th St E

Stewart Field

27th St W

35

27th St E

28th St W

0   300   600   900 yards

0   300   600   900 meters

29th St W

4 NICOLLET AVENUE'S EAT STREET: WHERE THE TWIN CITIES EAT GLOBAL LOCALLY

BOUNDARIES: 29th St. W., Nicollet Ave., Grant St. W.
HUDSON'S TWIN CITY STREET ATLAS **COORDINATES: Map 394, 2C and 2D**
DISTANCE: Approx. 2¾ miles
DIFFICULTY: Easy
PARKING: Free parking on 25th St.; free parking (2 hours or less) on Nicollet Ave.
PUBLIC TRANSIT: Bus lines 4, 113, and 115

Eat Street is Minneapolis's culinary connection to the world, boasting 17 city blocks of restaurants, markets, and coffee shops with food from around the world. It's a destination for both novices and experienced foodies in search of toothsome adventures. Nicollet Ave. cuts through three neighborhoods—most prominently Whittier, once an affluent area that fell into dilapidation in the '70s in the wake of the wealthy moving to the suburbs and the construction of I-35 W. Immigrants from mostly Asia—and later the Middle East, Europe, Mexico, and Africa—converted a wide array of buildings into restaurants. Over time it has become the incredible all-American ethnic food area known as Eat Street.

For this walk, bring a hearty appetite with you. The walk follows Nicollet Ave. to the outskirts of downtown Minneapolis and Loring Park, through Stevens Square, and back to Whittier. More than 55 businesses for eat-in or takeout food from around the world are located in this ever-changing whirlwind of a neighborhood. The area is always in transition, with new Americans taking language classes and participating in start-up businesses on the same street, while new condos and chain businesses keep moving in. Take a walk and see Minneapolis's gateway to world cuisine in the scenic shadows of downtown.

● Start at the corner of 25th St. W. and Nicollet Ave. in front of hipster and artist hangout Spyhouse Espresso Bar and Gallery. Cross 25th St. W. and head north up Nicollet Ave.

● Continue forward, crossing 24th St. W. The next few blocks are home to several schools that teach English as a second language for both children and adults, including the English Language Immersion School and the Somali Education Center. Up

ahead are nonfood-related ethnic businesses such as hair salons and financial planning businesses, as well as apartments and recent cookie-cutter condo developments
with national chain franchises at street level.

After you cross Franklin Ave., Eat Street enters the Loring Park neighborhood. Cross
18th St. W. and go straight. From here, you can see the perpetual transition that is Eat
Street, where vacant lots sit beside both fledgling and well-established businesses,
all in close proximity to the downtown skyline. Since the beginning of the new millen-
nium, condos have become increasingly common.

● Turn left at the corner of Grant St. W., and then immediately turn left again to follow
Nicollet Ave., past a block of condos. The next block has high-quality restaurants,
including the legendary Market Bar-B-Que (barbecue baby back ribs and Texas beef
ribs). Another block ahead, on the right, is Jerusalem's Restaurant, which offers tasty
Middle Eastern combos along with weekend belly dancing.

● Cross 18th St. W. and you'll come to the Plymouth Congregational Church (1908), a
Gothic Revival church made of granite and limestone trim. Just past Franklin Ave. on
the right-hand side is the Art Deco sign of Franklin-Nicollet Liquor, especially cool-
looking when illuminated in the evening.

● Cross 25th St. W. and go straight, passing an exciting assortment of restaurants and
ethnic grocery stores, as well as Icehouse Restaurant, an innovative nightclub from
the owners of Be'Wiched.

● Cross 26th St. W. Peninsula Malaysian Cuisine offers delicious authentic food from a
nation where Chinese, Malaysian, and Indian food traditions have combined for cen-
turies to create outstanding polyglot dishes such as roti *canai,* fish in banana leaf,
and beef *rendang.* Continue forward, crossing 29th St. W. Near the end of the street
is access to the Midtown Greenway—a pedestrian- and bicycle-only path connecting
Uptown and the lakes to the W. River Pkwy.

● Turn left at the end of the street and then left again, returning in the opposite direction on Nicollet Ave. Pho Tau Bay serves, as the sign says, "the best soup in town,"
and includes a full Vietnamese menu that even the parsimonious can afford.

- Continue forward, crossing 28th St. W. On the right is Rainbow Chinese Restaurant and Bar. Since 1987, chef and owner Tammy Wong has provided fresh and inventive fine Chinese food. On the next block is local favorite Quang, which features tasty Vietnamese cuisine. The next local favorite is the Black Forest Inn, which has served excellent German food including sauerbraten, schnitzel, and bratwurst—best washed down with beer—for more than 40 years. In the summertime, you can dine outside in the beautifully designed Beer Garden, a charming natural oasis secluded on the busy street by trees, shrubs, flowers, and a fountain.

- Cross 26th St. W. Up the block at 2539 Nicollet Ave. is Pancho Villa Restaurant, specializing in outstanding seafood and authentic Mexican food. The address was the longtime home of Twin/Tone Records, the label for local indie stalwarts such as the Replacements and Soul Asylum. The address, then 2541, became the title of a great song on Grant Hart's first post–Hüsker Dü solo album, *Intolerance*.

- Continue to the corner of 25th St. W. to finish the walk.

POINTS OF INTEREST

Spyhouse Espresso Bar and Gallery spyhousecoffeeshop.com, 2451 Nicollet Ave., Minneapolis, MN 55404, 612-871-3177

Market Bar-B-Que marketbbq.com, 1414 Nicollet Ave., Minneapolis, MN 55403, 612-872-1111

Jerusalem's Restaurant 1518 Nicollet Ave., Minneapolis, MN 55403, 612-871-8883

Plymouth Congregational Church plymouth.org, 1900 Nicollet Ave., Minneapolis, MN 55403, 612-871-7400

Icehouse Restaurant icehousempls.com, 2528 Nicollet Ave., Minneapolis, MN 55404, 612-276-6523

Peninsula Malaysian Cuisine peninsulamalaysiancuisine.com, 2608 Nicollet Ave., Minneapolis, MN 55408, 612-871-8282

Pho Tau Bay photaubay.us, 2837 Nicollet Ave., Minneapolis, MN 55408, 612-874-6030

Rainbow Chinese Restaurant and Bar rainbowrestaurant.com, 2739 Nicollet Ave., Minneapolis, MN 55403, 612-870-7081

Quang quangrestaurant.com, 2719 Nicollet Ave., Minneapolis, MN 55408, 612-874-6030

Black Forest Inn blackforestinnmpls.com, 1 26th St. E., Minneapolis, MN 55404, 612-872-0812

Pancho Villa Restaurant panchovillasgrill.com, 2539 Nicollet Ave., Minneapolis, MN 55404, 612-871-7014

route Summary

1. Start at the corner of 25th St. W. and Nicollet Ave. Cross 25th St. to follow Nicollet Ave.
2. Continue forward to the corner of Grant St. W. and turn left.
3. Immediately turn left again to follow Nicollet Ave. in the opposite direction.
4. Continue forward after crossing 18th St. W.
5. At the end of the street, turn left and left again, returning in the opposite direction on Nicollet Ave.
6. Continue to the corner of 25th St. W. to finish the walk.

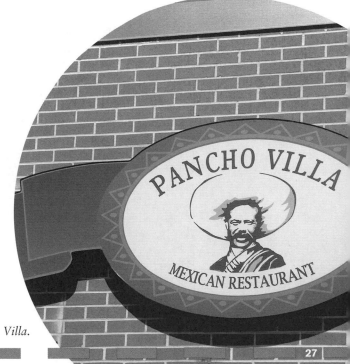

For authentic Mexican fare, try Pancho Villa.

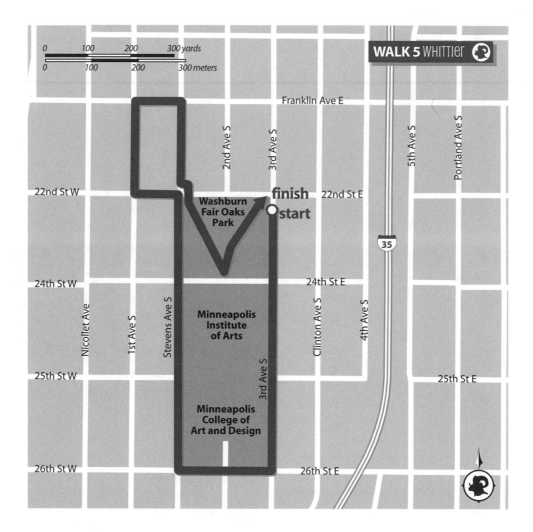

0 100 200 300 yards
0 100 200 300 meters

Franklin Ave E

2nd Ave S

3rd Ave S

5th Ave S

Portland Ave S

22nd St W

finish
start

22nd St E

Washburn
Fair Oaks
Park

24th St W

24th St E

Nicollet Ave

1st Ave S

Stevens Ave S

**Minneapolis
Institute
of Arts**

Clinton Ave S

4th Ave S

35

25th St W

3rd Ave S

25th St E

**Minneapolis
College of
Art and Design**

26th St W

26th St E

5 WHITTIER: MIA & WASHBURN FAIR OAKS: ART & NATURE COME ALIVE

BOUNDARIES: 26th St. E., 1st Ave. S., Franklin Ave. E., 3rd Ave. S.
HUDSON'S TWIN CITY STREET ATLAS **COORDINATES: Map 394, 2C and 2D**
DISTANCE: Approx. 1½ miles
DIFFICULTY: Easy
PARKING: Free parking on 22nd St. E.
PUBLIC TRANSIT: Bus lines 2, 5, 17, and 580

The Whittier neighborhood walk connects the past with the present via the principle source of wealth in Minneapolis's early days: flour. The mansions, Washburn Fair Oaks Park, and even the Minneapolis Institute of Arts (MIA) are all the beneficiaries of the affluence created by the Mill Cities' founders. They moved here, far south of downtown, to escape the grimy and filthy Mississippi River. Early in the 20th century, the urban blight they left behind had caught up with them—and the majority of the wealthy moved farther from the city's core. No longer strictly a bastion of the well-to-do, Whittier is home to a diverse group of immigrants, working class, middle class, young people, artists, and, of course, the few residents remaining in historic mansions.

● **Begin on the southwest corner of 22nd St. E. and go south on 3rd Ave. S. On the right is Washburn Fair Oaks Park, the former site of William Washburn's enormous stone mansion until 1924. After making his fortune in the flour-milling industry at St. Anthony Falls, he was elected to the U.S. House of Representatives and later to the U.S. Senate. On the left is the Gothic and Renaissance–inspired Hennepin History Museum. Originally the George H. and Leonora Christian House (George was an early manager of the Washburn Crosby Company, which later became General Mills), it now serves as the home of the Hennepin County History Society.**

● **Continue forward, crossing 24th St. E. On the right is the rather prosaic modernist 1974 addition to the Minneapolis Institute of Arts. Connected to the entrance is the Children's Theatre Company, expanded with a kid-friendly design by architect Michael Graves in 2005. Across the street are fine examples of the Colonial Revival** style, the Fair Oaks Apartments (1940). The one- and two-bedroom apartments are complemented by courtyards and lush gardens.

● After passing the Children's Theatre, continue on 3rd Ave. S. The 2500 block was the location of the Dorilus Morrison House (1858), home to the first mayor of Minneapolis. The building was razed to make room for the south portion of MIA in 1915.

● Turn right on 26th St. E. This section of Whittier is a modest residential area for hipsters. Continuing on 26th St., you'll see the back of Minneapolis College of Art and Design (MCAD). Since 1974 it has provided an excellent fine-arts education and now has more than 700 students.

● Turn right on Stevens Ave. S. To the right is MCAD's main entrance, complete with sculptures. Across the street are fine examples of quirkily renovated Victorian homes, with superbly unusual color combinations. Up ahead and on the right is the 2006 addition by Michael Graves, the aforementioned architect and Target product designer. The addition dovetails with the former MIA structure, and the added gallery space is especially welcome.

● Continue on Stevens Ave. S. At 24th St. E. is Washburn Fair Oaks Park.

MIA: Art Through the Ages Without the Price of Admission

The Minneapolis Institute of Arts (MIA) has a staggering art collection in terms of depth and especially breadth—name a period, style, or form, and it is represented. From Romanticism, Impressionism, and Judaica to photography, Pop Art, and Prairie School architecture and design, MIA has a tremendous scope of art that includes 100,000 pieces from 5,000 years of history. The museum expanded from its fledgling beginning in 1883 as the Minneapolis Society of Fine Arts with the construction of two additions in 1915. The range of art in the museum is immense, and because admission to the museum is free (with donations suggested), visitors can leisurely examine periods, styles, and techniques specific to their interests. The D'Amico-managed ArtsBreak coffee shop and Artscafe Restaurant offer an opportunity to lounge, while the family area provides a place for kids to play with hands-on activities that offer a slight artistic bent.

- Cross 22nd St. E., where you can view the Beaux Arts perfection known as the Gale Mansion (1912) on the corner (at 2115 Stevens Ave. S.). With its lovely Renaissance Revival–inspired features, it stands out as an architectural gem.

- Turn left on 22nd St. E. for a closer look at the mansions that define the area, such as the Alfred F. Pillsbury House (116 22nd St. E.), a huge Tudor Revival constructed with local limestone. Alfred was the son of John Pillsbury, who founded the world-famous food company. The next home is another Tudor Revival, originally built for milling mogul Charles S. Pillsbury, nephew of John Pillsbury; since 1993 the home has served as the offices for BLIND, Inc. (at 100 22nd St. E.).

- Turn right on 1st Ave. S. The Institute for Agricultural and Trade Policy, a Georgian Revival–style building, appears on the right. The lovely brick house was built by notable local architect William Channing Whitney for Caroline Crosby, daughter of a founder of the company that later became General Mills. Across the street at the corner are nondescript neo-traditional condos that recently replaced a gas station on this site.

- Turn right on Franklin Ave. E., and take a look at the downtown Minneapolis skyline.

- Turn right on Stevens Ave. S. and continue down the block, where you'll see a wide array of housing stock on this block, ranging from modest to turn-of-the-century luxurious.

- Cross 22nd St. E., and enter Washburn Fair Oaks Park. Proceed on the immediate diagonal path and enjoy the fresh air or take a seat on one of the many park benches.

- Continue straight at the fork in the path.

  The path terminates at 24th St. E., where the splendor of the original 1916 MIA can be enjoyed in proper perspective: a fine example of Classic Revival designed by the then-influential New York architecture firm of McKim, Mead, and White. The entrance stands out with its striking Ionian portico, which is completed with angels and Classic Chinese lions.

- Turn around and follow the northeast path back to the start/finish point at 22nd St. E. and 3rd Ave. S.

POINTS OF INTEREST

Washburn Fair Oaks Park tinyurl.com/wfopark, 200 24th St. E., Minneapolis, MN 55405, 612-230-6400

Hennepin History Museum hennepinhistory.org, 2303 3rd Ave. S., Minneapolis, MN 55404, 612-870-1329

Minneapolis Institute of Arts artsmia.org, 2400 3rd Ave. S., Minneapolis, MN 55404, 612-870-3132

The Children's Theatre Company childrenstheatre.org, 2400 3rd Ave. S., Minneapolis, MN 55404, 612-874-0400

Minneapolis College of Art and Design mcad.edu, 2501 Stevens Ave. S., Minneapolis, MN, 55404, 612-874-3700

ROUTE SUMMARY

1. Begin on the southwest corner of 22nd St. E. and go south on 3rd Ave. S.
2. Cross 24th St. E.
3. After passing the Children's Theatre, continue on 3rd Ave S.
4. Turn right on 26th St. E.
5. Turn right on Stevens Ave. S.
6. Cross, and then turn left on 22nd St. E.
7. Turn right on 1st Ave S.
8. Turn right on Franklin Ave. E.
9. Turn right on Stevens Ave. S.
10. Cross 22nd St. E., and enter Washburn Fair Oaks Park.
11. Continue south at the fork in the path.
12. The path terminates at 24th St. E. Turn around and follow the northeast path back to the start/finish point at 22nd St. E. and 3rd Ave. S.

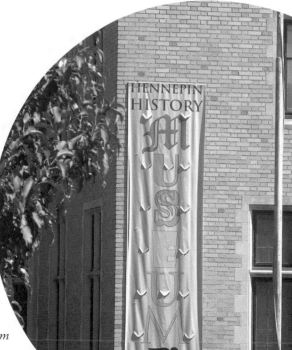

Hennepin History Museum

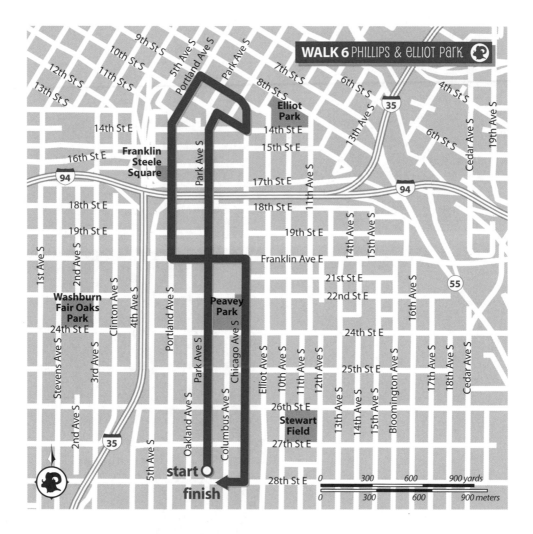

WALK 6 PHILLIPS & ELLIOT PARK

9th St S
10th St S
11th St S
12th St S
13th St S
14th St E
16th St E
18th St E
19th St E
24th St E
Franklin Steele Square
Washburn Fair Oaks Park
Peavey Park
Stewart Field
Elliot Park
5th Ave S
Portland Ave S
Park Ave S
7th St S
8th St S
6th St S
4th St S
19th Ave S
Cedar Ave S
13th Ave S
6th St S
14th St E
15th St E
17th St E
18th St E
19th St E
Franklin Ave E
11th Ave S
14th Ave S
15th Ave S
21st St E
22nd St E
24th St E
25th St E
26th St E
27th St E
28th St E
16th Ave S
Park Ave S
Portland Ave S
Park Ave S
Chicago Ave S
Oakland Ave S
Columbus Ave S
Elliot Ave S
10th Ave S
11th Ave S
12th Ave S
13th Ave S
14th Ave S
15th Ave S
Bloomington Ave S
17th Ave S
18th Ave S
Cedar Ave S
1st Ave S
2nd Ave S
Clinton Ave S
4th Ave S
Stevens Ave S
3rd Ave S
2nd Ave S
5th Ave S

94
35
94
35
55

start
finish

0   300   600   900 yards
0   300   600   900 meters

6 PHILLIPS & ELLIOT PARK: Park Avenue Urban Shape Shifter

BOUNDARIES: **28th St. E., Portland Ave. S., 9th St. S., Chicago Ave. S.**
HUDSON'S TWIN CITY STREET ATLAS COORDINATES: **Map 394, 3C and 3D**
DISTANCE: **Approx. 3½ miles**
DIFFICULTY: **Easy**
PARKING: **Free parking on Park Ave. S.**
PUBLIC TRANSIT: **Bus lines 5 and 11**

Park Avenue conjures up images of the affluent street of the same name in New York City, and elsewhere across the United States where the name was given to neighborhoods in obvious imitation. The Park Ave. area of Minneapolis was once the city's Victorian mansion row—much as Summit Ave. is in St. Paul, with more than 30 mansions between 18th and 28th Streets. However, Park Ave. suffered a different fate than Summit Ave. due to its easily accessible location directly south of downtown on flat prairie land. Instead of falling into disrepair and remaining so for decades, as its larger St. Paul counterpart did, Park Ave. was repeatedly redeveloped from 1890 to its 1920 heyday. Numerous great mansions on Park Ave. were razed, carved into apartments, or converted into homes for organizations such as the Ebenezer Church offices, the Shriners (Zuhrah Shrine Temple, 2540 Park Ave.), and social organizations such as chemical-dependency halfway houses and mental health treatment centers. The remaining Park Ave. mansions are most heavily concentrated in the Phillips neighborhood, while the north part of the walk heads into the Elliot Park neighborhood in the shadow of downtown. After losing almost half its population to freeway construction between 1950 and 1970, Elliot Park, today more affluent than Phillips, has become a hip hub for renovated and newly constructed apartments and condos.

● **Begin at the corner of 28th St. E. and Park Ave. S. Observe the odd mixture of architecture that includes mansions, apartments, and functional corporate and organization buildings, such as the Ebenezer Corporate Offices and Park Apartments.**

● **Head north on Park Ave., crossing 27th St. E. Across the street is a local landmark and important cultural institution: the American Swedish Institute (ASI). The gaudy**

Châteauesque and Baroque Revival beauty was constructed in 1908 for Swan J. Turnblad, publisher of the *Svenska Amerikanska Posten,* then the largest-selling Swedish-language newspaper in America. In 2012 ASI added the Nelson Cultural Center, featuring a gallery, an event center, a classroom offering Swedish language and craft classes, and a new museum shop. The jewel of the new space is the café, Fika, which offers a selection of Swedish-inspired, reasonably priced gourmet cuisine.

- Cross 26th St. E. On the left corner is the Zuhrah Shrine Temple (1902), a lovely Italian Renaissance Revival mansion. Many old mansions here have been converted for new purposes, such as the various psychotherapy practices at Park Avenue Center and, across the street, the prosaic institutional buildings of St. Mary's University campus that fill more than two blocks.

- Cross 25th St. E. On the right is Lemna Technologies (2445 Park Ave. S.). The building was originally the home of Anson and Georgia Brooks, who made their fortune in lumber but lived in a striking Venetian Gothic–style stone mansion.

- Cross 24th St. E. On the right is where the greatest number of Victorian mansions for high-society Minneapolitans—including the home of James Ford Bell, the longtime head of General Mills—were demolished. Across the street are two mansions serving a new purpose. The Renaissance Revival George Peavey House (2222 Park Ave. S.) is now known as Freeport West, Inc. The neighboring, colossal Romanesque Revival–style Sumner and Eugenie McKnight House (2200 Park Ave. S.) is currently occupied by American Indian Services.

- Cross Franklin Ave. E., an area that was marred by drug dealers during the '80s and '90s but has made a comeback in recent years due to diligent efforts and collaboration of local residents and the Minneapolis Police Department. On the left is Straitgate Church, a massive brownstone church formerly known as Park Avenue Congregational.

- Continue straight on Park Ave. S., crossing the bridge over I-94, which provides an alluring vantage point for downtown Minneapolis and the Elliot Park neighborhood in the immediate foreground. The next few blocks are in a state of flux as condos and redevelopment encroach; there are few single-family homes in this predominantly high-density, mixed-use area.

- After crossing 14th St. E., follow Park Ave. S. (Frontage Rd.) as it curves slightly to the right next to the redbrick Drexel Apartment Hotel.

- Turn right on 10th St. S. Ahead is a nice section of the neighborhood filled with businesses, condos, and apartments.

- Turn left on 14th St. E. On the corner is the Band Box Diner. During the 1920s, the automobile became attainable for middle-income families and made possible this precursor to modern fast-food restaurants. The diner, which opened in 1929, mimicked the White Castle chain, serving inexpensive burgers and fries. One of 14 locations at the time, it sat vacant for years before reopening in 2003 to serve casual American fare.

- Turn left on the corner of 14th St. E. to follow Chicago Ave. S., enjoying the spectacular view of downtown.

- Continue on Chicago Ave. S., crossing Centennial Pl., where five city streets converge on the grid, and turn left on 9th St. S. This street contains several of the city's most beautiful apartments, such as the Rappahannock—a huge stone apartment with wrought iron balconies, constructed in 1895.

- Turn left on Portland Ave. S. This section of Elliot Park combines newly constructed and renovated condos. On the left are the Skyscape Condos.

Band Box Diner

SWAN J. TURNBLAD: THE AMERICAN DREAM SWEDISH-STYLE & THE FOUNDING OF THE AMERICAN SWEDISH INSTITUTE

Swan J. Turnblad was the embodiment of the Swedish American version of the American Dream. Born in rural Sweden, the youngest of 11 children, he immigrated in 1868 as a small child with his family to Vasa Township, the early Swedish settlement south of the Twin Cities. In 1879 he moved to Minneapolis, where he quickly rose as an important editor and publisher of Swedish-language newspapers, most notably the *Svenska Amerikanska Posten*. He purchased stock for the first issue in 1885, and by 1888 he owned and published the paper. Under his leadership, the circulation grew from a faltering national Swedish-language paper to the undisputed leader by the 1890s. Even more important, by 1890 the number of Swedish immigrants in the US had doubled from a decade before to 478,000, with 21%

living in Minnesota. Turnblad also engaged in real estate speculation, in part to buy property to develop a family home.

In 1903 he purchased six lots at 2600 Park Ave., where he would construct his enormous castlelike dream home, completed in 1908. Turnblad astutely realized that the Swedish-language demographic was aging, Americanizing, and shrinking, and he sold his newspaper in 1920. Turnblad died a few years later, but the organization he founded would become an astounding local and national success, with exhibits and other cultural events celebrating Swedish culture. In 2008 the former Turnblad mansion celebrated its 100th anniversary, and in 2012 the American Swedish Institute expanded to accommodate additional gallery space and a restaurant.

- Continue on Portland Ave. S., crossing 10th St. S., an area lined with a collection of solid renovations, such as the Balmoral Apartments, and garish new constructions.

- Cross 16th St. E. On the right is Franklin Steele Square. The small park was a gift from the daughters of the pioneer Steele—a pivotal leader in the early history of the community that was annexed in 1872 by Minneapolis.

- Cross I-94 and return to the Phillips neighborhood. Again, this area has improved over the past decade, but many homes are in need of renovation.

- Cross 19th St. E. On the left is St. Paul's Evangelical Lutheran Church, a Romanesque Revival gem constructed of brownstone and granite in 1889, and originally a Presbyterian church. The next block was once a haven for illegal drug sales and use. After demolition, some of the property has remained vacant, while condos and affordable apartments have been constructed on other lots.

- Turn left at the corner of Franklin Ave. E.

- Turn right on Chicago Ave. S. On the left a few blocks down at 15th St. E. was a tiny Romanian Jewish district at the turn of the century until after World War II. On the right is Peavey Park, with sculptures and an abundance of park benches.

- Continue south on Chicago Ave. S., where the new Minneapolis Grand Apartments are across the street from condemned and dilapidated homes.

- Cross 25th St. E. On the left is the cheery architecture of Children's Hospitals and Clinics, which stands in stark contrast to the drab institutional look of the hospitals ahead.

- Cross 27th St. E. to walk through a neighborhood of huge, well-maintained Victorians.

- Cross 28th St. E. and turn right; then walk to the finish point at 28th St. and Park Ave.

POINTS OF INTEREST

American Swedish Institute/Fika asimn.org, 2600 Park Ave. S., Minneapolis, MN 55407, 612-871-4907

St. Mary's University smumn.edu, 2500 Park Ave., Minneapolis, MN 55404, 612-728-5100

Straitgate Church straitgate.org, 638 Franklin Ave. E., Minneapolis, MN 55404, 612-870-7472

Band Box Diner facebook.com/bandboxeats, 729 10th St. S., Minneapolis, MN 55404, 612-332-0850

Franklin Steele Square tinyurl.com/steelesquare, 1600 Portland Ave. S., Minneapolis, MN 55404, 612-230-6400

St. Paul's Evangelical Lutheran Church stpaulsevlutheran.org, 1901 Portland Ave. S., Minneapolis, MN 55404, 612-874-0133

Peavey Park tinyurl.com/peaveypark, 730 22nd St. E., Minneapolis, MN 55404, 612-230-6400

ROUTE SUMMARY

1. Begin at the corner of 28th Ave. E. and Park Ave. S.
2. Head north on Park Ave. S., crossing 27th St. E.
3. After crossing 14th St. E., follow Park Ave. S. (Frontage Rd.) as it curves slightly to the right.
4. Turn right on 10th St. S.
5. Cross 10th St. S. and turn left on 14th St. E.
6. Turn left at 14th St. E. and onto Chicago Ave. S.
7. Continue on Chicago Ave. S., crossing Centennial Pl., where five city streets converge on the grid, and turn left on 9th St. S.
8. Turn left on Portland Ave. S.
9. Turn left on Franklin Ave. E.
10. Turn right on Chicago Ave. S.
11. Cross 28th St. E. and turn right, returning to the starting point at 28th St. E. and Park Ave. S.

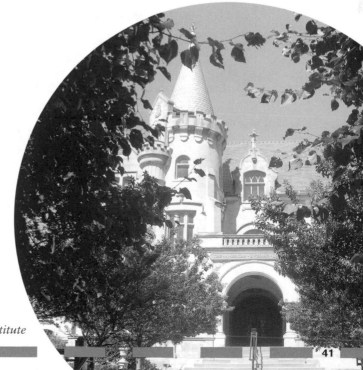

American Swedish Institute

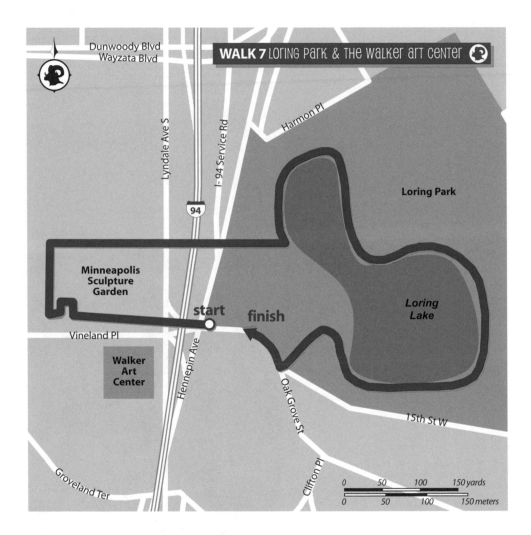

Dunwoody Blvd
Wayzata Blvd

Lyndale Ave S

I-94 Service Rd

94

Harmon Pl

Loring Park

Minneapolis
Sculpture
Garden

Loring
Lake

start finish

Vineland Pl

Walker
Art
Center

Hennepin Ave

Oak Grove St

15th St W

Groveland Ter

Clifton Pl

0   50   100   150 yards
0   50   100   150 meters

7 LorInG Park & THe Walker arT CenTer: arT & NaTure aT a NeXus

BOUNDARIES: **Oak Grove St., Vineland Pl., Dunwoody Blvd., Harmon Pl., Willow St., 15th St. W.**
HUDSON'S TWIN CITY STREET ATLAS COORDINATES: **Map 394, 1C and 2C**
DISTANCE: **Approx. 1 mile**
DIFFICULTY: **Easy**
PARKING: **2-hour metered parking on Willow St.; paid parking at the Walker Art Center Parking Ramp on Vineland Pl.**
PUBLIC TRANSIT: **Bus lines 17 and 18**

Loring Park and the Walker Art Center seamlessly integrate artsy aesthetic with earthy utilitarianism. This is the place for contemporary art in all media, as well as the place for reflecting on and basking in the wealth of nature. Despite its geographic shortcomings—several major roads bisect the park and the art center—the beauty of the area's architecture and green space supplant the nearby freeway's din. The Irene Hixon Whitney Bridge (1988) is a crucial element in creating this environment—it crosses 16 lanes of traffic; yet the pedestrian and bicycle span provides a panoramic view of the exquisite surroundings, while linking the park and the works of art. Both institutions are rooted in Minneapolis's early rise to national prominence; the Walker Art Center takes its name from a local lumberman turned art collector and philanthropist, Thomas Walker. His original museum was constructed near the present-day site in 1927, but it was replaced with the much larger modernist structure by Edward Barnes Larrabee in 1971. Then in 2005, the Walker expanded again—this time, noted Swiss architects Jacques Herzog and Pierre de Meuron added 130,000 square feet along Hennepin Ave.

Loring Park has an equally important history in Minneapolis: it opened in 1883 as Central Park. It was modeled on the world-famous park of the same name in New York City—despite the fact that the name of Minneapolis's version was a misnomer because it is central to nothing in the city. The 35-acre park and the picturesque lake (formerly Johnson Lake) were later renamed in honor of flour-milling magnate and the city's first park board commissioner, Charles Loring. To complement the artistic, natural, and civil-engineered beauty, the area has an abundance of moderately priced fine-dining establishments—many with alfresco patios and rooftop tables during warm-weather months.

● Begin at the northeast corner of Oak Grove St. and Hennepin Ave. Looking up the hill to the left, you'll see two of the finest examples of church architecture in the city, both designed by Minneapolis architect Edwin Hewitt. Immediately across the street on the left is St. Mark's Episcopal Cathedral (1911). Hewitt was a member of this parish, and the building was inspired by English Gothic style and Magdalen College at Oxford. St. Mark's began as a parish church but was elevated to a cathedral in 1941. Farther up Hennepin Ave. is the 238-foot spire of Hennepin Avenue United Methodist Church. The Gothic-inspired church was designed in 1916 by Hewitt and his brother-in-law.

Between the two churches are the 510 Groveland Apartments; the Renaissance Revival building now houses condos and a nationally recognized elegant restaurant, La Belle Vie. The fine, eclectic, Mediterranean-influenced menu has received countless accolades, including a nod as one of America's Top 50 Restaurants in *Gourmet* magazine in 2006. Another perspective that highlights the magnitude of the architecture on this block is from the Irene Hixon Whitney Bridge.

● Continue straight, carefully crossing Hennepin Ave. and Lyndale Ave. Across the street is the Walker Art Center: a national leader in contemporary visual

THE MINNEAPOLIS SCULPTURE GARDEN: FINE ART IN THE OUTSIDE ENVIRONMENT

The Twin Cities provide a wealth of opportunities for appreciating the intersection of nature and art: the Minneapolis Sculpture Garden is the best exemplar. Comprising 40 permanent works of art—even before the planned expansion—the museum's art, arbor, bridge, and conservatory are on view thanks to the collaboration between the Walker Art Center and the Minneapolis Park Board. Of course, the most well-known public art is *Spoonbridge and Cherry* (1985–89) by husband and wife Pop Art sculptors Claes Oldenburg and Coosje Van Bruggen. Another notable work is *Standing Frame*, a wood frame created by environmental artist David Nash. Then there's Charles Ginnever's enormous steel minimalist sculpture, *Nautilus*, which resembles a massive mollusk of the same name. The sculpture garden, which opened in 1988, has plans to expand on the 4-acre site that formerly featured Tyrone Guthrie Theater, planned by the late University of Minnesota architect and professor Ralph Rapson.

and performing arts. The Walker exhibits a diverse permanent collection as well as traveling exhibitions, which have included works by Frida Kahlo and Pablo Picasso. In addition, dance, films, music, and classes are available at the august art institution. The Walker's restaurant, Gather, features a different, highly esteemed chef every month and is operated by Wolfgang Puck. The restaurant is located above Hennepin Ave. and offers an amazing view of the city, perfect for savoring Asian-influenced California cuisine.

- At the second set of stairs between the paired pillars, go down the stairs and then enter at the MINNEAPOLIS SCULPTURE GARDEN sign. The profusion of sculptures in the 11½-acre free public sculpture gallery is staggering and worthy of hours of examination.

- Turn left at the first pathway intersection, and then turn left again at the entrance to the Cowles Conservatory, redolent with flowers.

- Continue straight through the conservatory. In the center is *Standing Glass Fish,* an enormous 22-foot-tall sculpture of glass, wood, rubber, steel, and plexiglass by architect Frank Gehry.

- Turn right after exiting the conservatory and continue straight toward *Spoonbridge and Cherry,* the most recognizable piece of public art in the Twin Cities.

- After viewing the sculpture garden, continue toward the Irene Hixon Whitney Bridge.

- Cross the bridge toward Loring Park. The bridge provides an incredible scenic vista above Hennepin Ave. On the right, you can see the first part of the walk, as well as downtown Minneapolis, the Walker Art Center, and Loring Park, from a unique perspective. On the left is the nearby Basilica of Saint Mary, an enormous Beaux Arts procathedral (or secondary cathedral) for the Archdiocese of St. Paul and Minneapolis.

- Follow the stairs down to the innermost path at Loring Lake and turn left. Across the street from the park on the left is the Fawkes Building, originally an auto dealership 1911–1917. Today, it's home to several restaurants and businesses, including the upscale comfort-food restaurant Café Lurcat.

- Turn left near the lake, where you can perch on a park bench and observe the ducks, geese, orioles, cattails, and reeds in this natural environment surrounded by a quaint urban setting.

- Follow the curve around the lake. On the left are additional Loring Park businesses, featuring another fine restaurant with outdoor dining: Joe's Garage is a casual dining establishment with a bistro menu that includes burgers, fries, pastas, soups, and sandwiches, not to mention a splendid rooftop view.

- Continue on, passing the gardens and the bridge as the path veers to the left. The landscape architecture is stunning with the benches and flowers arranged in a circle—each bench provides another panoramic vantage point of the city. Follow the path along the irregular shape of the lake as it curves slightly to the right.

- Turn right as the path continues past the basketball court, playground, and the Mission Revival–style Loring Park Community Center (1906), all on the left.

- Turn right at the bend and follow the contour of the lake. On the left across 15th St. are several beautiful pieces of architecture, including the rear of the Renaissance Revival–style Woman's Club of Minneapolis (1927), which continues to host lectures and concerts here.

- Turn left at the fork in the path. Then turn right and proceed to finish the walk at the intersection of Hennepin Ave. and Oak Grove St.

POINTS OF INTEREST

St. Mark's Episcopal Cathedral ourcathedral.org, 519 Oak Grove St., Minneapolis, MN 55403, 612-870-7800

Hennepin Avenue United Methodist Church hennepinchurch.org, 511 Groveland Ave., Minneapolis, MN 55403, 612-871-5303

La Belle Vie labellevie.us, 510 Groveland Ave., Minneapolis, MN 55403, 612-874-6440

Walker Art Center walkerart.org, 1750 Hennepin Ave., Minneapolis, MN 55403, 612-375-7622

Gather gatherbydamico.com, 1750 Hennepin Ave., Minneapolis, MN 55403, 612-253-3400

Basilica of Saint Mary mary.org, 88 17th St. N., Minneapolis, MN 55403, 612-333-1381

Café Lurcat cafelurcat.com, 1624 Harmon Pl., Minneapolis, MN 55403, 612-486-5500

Loring Park tinyurl.com/loringlake, 1382 Willow St., Minneapolis, MN 55403, 612-370-4929

Joe's Garage joes-garage.com, 1610 Harmon Pl., Minneapolis, MN 55403, 612-904-1163

Woman's Club of Minneapolis womansclub.org, 410 Oak Grove St., Minneapolis, MN 55403, 612-870-8001

route summary

1. Begin at the northeast corner of Oak Grove St. and Hennepin Ave.
2. Continue straight, carefully crossing Hennepin Ave. and Lyndale Ave.
3. At the second set of stairs between the pillars, go down the stairs and enter at the MINNEAPOLIS SCULPTURE GARDEN sign.
4. Turn left at the first pathway intersection, and turn left again at the entrance to the Cowles Conservatory.
5. Continue straight through the conservatory.
6. Then turn right after exiting the conservatory and continue toward *Spoonbridge and Cherry*.
7. Continue toward the Irene Hixon Whitney Bridge.
8. Cross the bridge to Loring Park.
9. After following the stairs straight down to the inner-most path next to Loring Lake, turn left.
10. Turn left near the lake, and follow the curve around the pond.
11. Continue on, passing the gardens and bridge as the path veers to the left.
12. Follow the path along the irregular shape of the lake.
13. Turn right as the path continues.
14. Turn right at the bend and follow the contour of the lake.
15. Turn left at the fork in the path, and then turn right to finish the walk at the intersection of Hennepin Ave. and Oak Grove St.

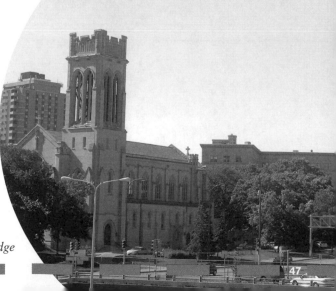

View from Irene Hixon Whitney Bridge

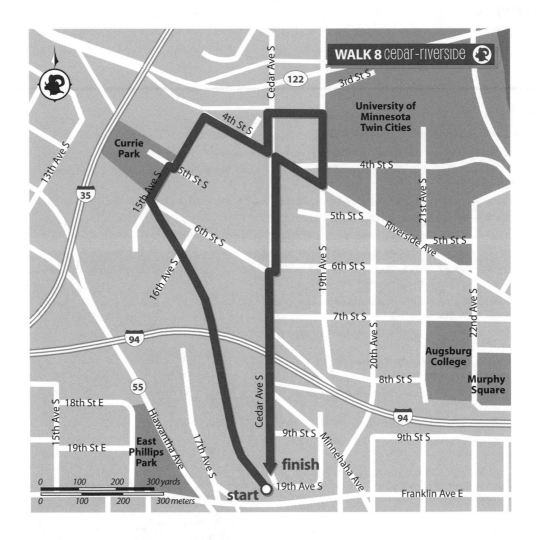

WALK 8 cedar-riverside

University of Minnesota Twin Cities

3rd St S

Cedar Ave S

4th St S

Currie Park

5th St S

15th Ave S

6th St S

16th Ave S

13th Ave S

35

94

55

15th Ave S

18th St E

19th St E

East Phillips Park

Hiawantha Ave

17th Ave S

Cedar Ave S

4th St S

5th St S

Riverside Ave

21st Ave S

5th St S

6th St S

19th Ave S

7th St S

20th Ave S

8th St S

22nd Ave S

Augsburg College

Murphy Square

94

9th St S

Minnehaha Ave

9th St S

start

finish

19th Ave S

Franklin Ave E

0   100   200   300 yards

0   100   200   300 meters

8 Cedar-Riverside: Ethnic Heritage Intersects With Counterculture

BOUNDARIES: Franklin Ave. E., Cedar Ave. S., 15th Ave. S., 3rd St. S., 19th Ave. S.
HUDSON'S TWIN CITY STREET ATLAS **COORDINATES: Map 394, 3C and 4C**
DISTANCE: Approx. 1¾ miles
DIFFICULTY: Easy
PARKING: 2-hour metered parking on 19th Ave. S. and Franklin Frontage Rd.; metered parking on Franklin Ave.
PUBLIC TRANSIT: Light-rail on the Hiawatha Line at Franklin Ave. Station

Cedar-Riverside has an enduring history as one of the Twin Cities' great ethnic salad bowls. It has also been an exemplar of a combined commercial and residential area, albeit for the working class or working poor, throughout each historic epoch. The triangle-shaped community is nestled between the Mississippi River, University of Minnesota, and two important interstate highways, I-35W and I-94. Diverse groups of people over the years have resided and shopped in the area sometimes referred to as the West Bank. Scandinavians dominated the neighborhood, particularly the business district on Cedar Ave., from the 1890s until the Great Depression. The neighborhood seriously declined after World War II. Large portions of its decaying housing were demolished to make room for interstate highways and the expansion of the University of Minnesota (U of M) on the west bank of the Mississippi River in the 1960s. The proximity to U of M and inexpensive housing inspired a burgeoning counterculture. The various modalities of the area's hippie past are readily apparent in the restaurants and stores—many originating from the early '70s punks, radicals, and reformers turned businesspeople. Since the early 1990s, immigrant groups, particularly the Somalis, have moved into the neighborhood's rental units and have created their own thriving businesses. The Cedar-Riverside community has become increasingly appealing because of its diversity—a neighborhood of old hippies, college kids, and recent immigrants—and easy accessibility by the Hiawatha Light-Rail Transit Line. Genuine counterculture and ongoing immigration history come alive on the streets of Cedar-Riverside.

● **Start at the Franklin Ave. Station and turn right on the combined pedestrian and bicycle path that runs parallel with the light-rail transit line.**

- Continue on this path and absorb the numerous scenic vistas of Minneapolis en route to the Cedar-Riverside Station. To the left is the light-rail transit garage, and just past I-94 is the colossal Riverside Plaza (1973), formerly Cedar Square West Apartments. The complex was part of the first federally supported urban New Town. Ralph Rapson, a University of Minnesota architecture professor, designed the modernist apartments—some with 1,300 apartment units that exceed 40 stories and stretch over 11 blocks. The slightly ominous structure experienced financial difficulties, suffered from bankruptcy, and was sold in the 1980s by the City of Minneapolis. The apartments are now home to numerous immigrants, especially Somalis.

- Cross the street at the crosswalk and turn right immediately on 15th Ave. S. On your left is Currie Park, I-35W, the Hubert H. Humphrey Metrodome, and downtown.

- Turn right on 5th St. S. and then turn left on 15th Ave. S. After passing the park, you'll see the Brian Coyle Community Center across the street. It serves the youth, families, and immigrants in the neighborhood. The building is named in honor of the late three-term Minneapolis city councilman, who was a strong advocate for human rights, housing, and the environment, as well as the rights of gay, lesbian, and transgender populations. Coyle died of AIDS in 1991.

- Turn right on 4th St. S. at the Mixed Blood Theatre, which was founded in 1976 by 22-year-old Jack Reuler. Since then it has produced a culturally pluralistic arts organization, though specializing in plays, in a renovated fire station.

- Turn left on Cedar Ave. S. Across the street is Midwest Mountaineering—the store for climbing, camping, paddling, travel, and all outdoors activities since 1970. The hippie-owned business moved to its present location in 1976 in the transitional counterculture hotbed, where it has expanded five times to better serve the outdoors adventurer.

- Turn right on 3rd St. S. Appropriately located down the stairs in Midwest Mountaineering's basement is Mayday Books, a volunteer collective nonprofit dedicated to selling progressive literature and magazines.

- Turn right on 19th Ave. S. Across the street is the University of Minnesota and its Hubert H. Humphrey Institute of Public Affairs and Carlson School of Management.

ceDar aVeNUe: MiNNeaPOLiS'S SNOOSe BOULeVarD

During its early history, Cedar-Riverside was one of America's great "Snoose Boulevards." It took its name from the teeming masses of Scandinavian immigrants who visited the area for the many social activities along Cedar Ave. S. from the 1890s until the early 20th century. "Snoose Boulevard" was a pejorative term coined by old-stock Americans aimed at denouncing the popular Scandinavian habit of chewing tobacco or snuset, especially by working men in the milling and lumber industries.

Built by the local Danish community, Dania Hall (1886) was the center of Scandinavian vaudeville and kept it thriving until the Depression. It would not recover as the Scandinavian population aged and moved from the neighborhood. The building was sold in 1963, and in 2000, after years of neglect and efforts to rebuild the landmark, it was destroyed by a fire.

Snoose Boulevard is in Cedar-Riverside's distant past, but the legacy continues in the waves of new immigrants living in the vast Riverside Plaza apartment buildings and walking Cedar Ave. today. The new, hardworking immigrants share the American Dream to improve their lives and those of their children, while shaping institutions and businesses in the neighborhood to serve their communities.

● Turn right on Riverside Ave. Across the street is the Hard Times Café, a cooperatively owned restaurant and coffee shop open 22 hours a day to serve members of the counterculture, from hippie to punk. On the right is the Bailey Building, home to KFAI (90.3 FM in Minneapolis or 106.7 FM in St. Paul), which provides community radio and a diverse voice for music and talk. On the corner is Acadia Café, recently relocated from Eat Street (Nicollet Ave.) to this large space. In the move, they've brought their eclectic nightly music schedule as well as a wide selection of tap beers (28!) plus coffee, burgers, and sandwiches.

● Turn left on Cedar Ave. S. Across the street is one of the Twin Cities' best dive restaurants—the Wienery, where they have perfected the art of the hot dog (including a tasty vegan version). The Cedar Cultural Center is a few doors down—the Twin Cities' premier venue for world music since 1991.

On the left is a vacant lot that used to house Dania Hall, the beloved site of Scandinavian vaudeville that was boarded up for years before burning down in 2000.

- Turn right after crossing 6th St. S., and turn left after crossing Cedar Ave. S. Up the block on Cedar Ave. S. is the Triple Rock Social Club, co-owned by Erik Funk of punk legends Dillinger Four. The club books the best in local and national music in a comfortable space with a wide selection of beer. The adjoining bar serves the best in bar food, including burgers, sandwiches, and an extensive vegetarian menu.

- Carefully walk under the I-94 overpass. On the right is the Community Peace Gardens.

- Continue to follow Cedar Ave. to the Franklin Ave. Station to finish the walk.

POINTS OF INTEREST

Currie Park tinyurl.com/mncurriepark, 500 15th Ave. S., Minneapolis, MN 55454, 612-230-6400

Mixed Blood Theatre mixedblood.com, 1501 4th St. S., Minneapolis, MN 55454, 612-338-0937

Midwest Mountaineering midwestmtn.com, 309 Cedar Ave. S., Minneapolis, MN 55454, 612-339-3433

Mayday Books maydaybookstore.org, 301 Cedar Ave. S., Minneapolis, MN 55454, 612-333-4719

University of Minnesota umn.edu/twincities, 321 19th Ave. S., Minneapolis, MN 55455, 612-625-2008

Hard Times Café hardtimes.com, 1821 Riverside Ave., Minneapolis, MN 55454, 612-341-9261

Acadia Café acadiacafe.com, 329 Cedar Ave. S., Minneapolis, MN 55454, 612-874-8702

The Wienery wienery.com, 414 Cedar Ave. S., Minneapolis, MN 55454, 612-333-5798

Cedar Cultural Center thecedar.org, 416 Cedar Ave. S., Minneapolis, MN 55454, 612-338-2674

Triple Rock Social Club triplerocksocialclub.com, 629 Cedar Ave. S., Minneapolis, MN 55454, 612-333-7399

Community Peace Gardens koreanservicemn.org/programs/prog_farm.php, 808 Cedar Ave. S., Minneapolis, MN 55454, 612-342-1344, ext. 5

route summary

1. Start at the Franklin Ave. Station and turn right, following the combined pedestrian/bicycle path running parallel with the light-rail transit line.

2. Continue on this path and absorb the numerous scenic vistas of Minneapolis en route to the Cedar-Riverside Station.

3. Cross the street at the crosswalk and turn right immediately on 15th Ave. S.

4. Turn right on 5th St. S. and then turn left on 15th Ave.

5. Turn right on 4th St. S. at the Mixed Blood Theatre.

6. Turn left on Cedar Ave. S.

7. Turn right on 3rd St. S.

8. Turn right on 19th Ave. S.

9. Turn right on Riverside Ave.

10. Turn left on Cedar Ave. S.

11. After crossing 6th St. S., turn right, and then turn left after crossing Cedar Ave. S.

12. Continue walking on Cedar Ave. S., carefully passing under I-94.

13. Continue walking to the Franklin Ave. Station to finish the walk.

You can see the sign for The Cabooze along the walk.

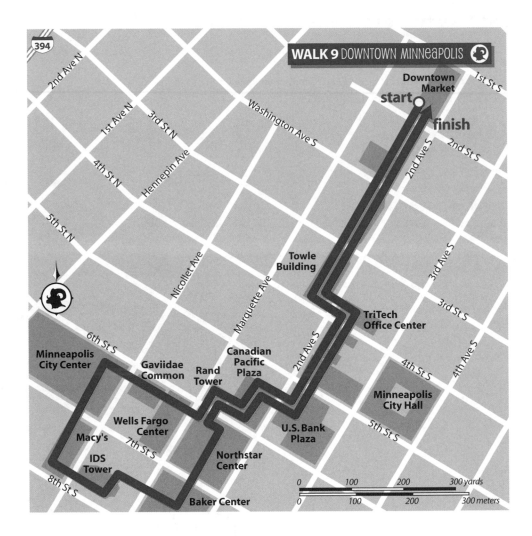

9 DOWNTOWN MINNEAPOLIS: FROM THE AIR

BOUNDARIES: 8th St. S., Hennepin Ave. S., 1st St. S., 3rd Ave. S.
HUDSON'S TWIN CITY STREET ATLAS **COORDINATES: Map 394, 2B and 3B**
DISTANCE: Approx. 1½ miles
DIFFICULTY: Easy
PARKING: Metered street parking on 2nd St. S.
PUBLIC TRANSIT: Bus lines 5, 9, 19, 22, and 24

In the middle of winter, when temperatures can get as low as -40°F, we Minneapolitans are thankful for every inch of the climate-controlled skyway system. These elevated walkways link 80 city blocks together and allow pedestrians and businesspeople to comfortably walk around downtown any time of year without a jacket. Built in the 1960s, Minneapolis's skyway system is more than 8 miles in length, the longest of its kind in the world. Almost every building in downtown Minneapolis with a street-level entrance will provide easy access to the skyway system Monday–Friday, with limited hours on weekends. During the summer months, fleets of food trucks can be seen congregating along Marquette Avenue between 7th and 8th Sts. through the skyway windows, any one of which is worth a trek down to the street level.

● Enter the Churchill building at 150 2nd Ave. S. Go past the Downtown Market and take the first left. Head up the stairs, go through the door at the top, and voilà! You've found the public access entrance to the Minneapolis downtown skyway system.

● Turn right and head straight into the skyway overpass. Here's your first aerial view of downtown Minneapolis, crossing Washington Ave. S. To your left, you'll see a panoramic view of Minneapolis's historic heart and the Milwaukee Road building with its distinctive clock tower, once a major stop for the great trains that rumbled through downtown until the mid-20th century.

● Head straight along the skyway and through the double doors at the end; now you're in The Crossings condominium building. Follow the path to the right.

● Go straight past the hanging sculptures and atrium overlook to get to the elevators at the far side of the building.

- Turn left at the elevators and go through the next skyway and into the Towle Building.

- Turn left at Tea House, an excellent Chinese restaurant offering an array of Szechuan specialties, and go out the doors and into the skyway that leads to the TriTech Office Center. For your convenience, a gigantic map of the entire skyway system is on the wall at the skyway entrance.

  When in the skyway, look left for a great view of the imposing Minneapolis City Hall building, complete with clock tower. You are now approaching the center of downtown Minneapolis.

- Follow the winding path through the TriTech building, past the escalator and straight ahead, until you get to the next skyway, which takes you to the Wells Fargo Midland Building. If you need a rest break, Classic Cookie sells great, huge cookies—they may be a little less like the homey goodness of your mom's cookies, but they're a whole lot fancier. Go around to the far end of the building and exit the skyway to your right.

  While in the skyway, make sure you stop to take in the city below you. You are now in the heart of downtown Minneapolis. On your left, you see the light-rail station, as well as the exterior of the CenturyLink Building, which you just exited. Behind you, the original Minnesota limestone–and–granite façade of the former Northwestern Bell Telephone Building is still completely intact, and is a sharp contrast to the ordinary-looking interior of this office building.

- Enter the U.S. Bank Plaza and turn right at the large, glowing map kiosk directly in front of you. Follow the path to the right to the next skyway into the Canadian Pacific Plaza building.

- Follow the path from the skyway past the escalators, turn right, and go down the short steps into the Rand Tower. Go straight until you reach the end of the hall, make a left, and exit the building into the skyway leading to the Northstar Center. Make sure that you check out the exterior of the Rand Tower from the skyway. It's an impressive building, constructed of Minnesota marble and granite and decorated with Art Deco flowers and leaves.

- Once in the Northstar Center, also called the Six Quebec building, go straight and turn right at Amy's Classic Confections, which carries an amazing selection of truffles from one of the best chocolatiers in the Twin Cities, if not the country: B. T. McElrath's. There should be a law that says you can't leave the Twin Cities without trying at least one B. T. McElrath's passion fruit truffle. Just past Amy's is the exit from the Northstar Center into the skyway.

- Go straight through the skyway. Directly below you is Nicollet Mall, a pedestrian, bike, and bus-only street, lined with restaurants and shops. The walls of this particular skyway sport stained glass panels that are fun for kids to peer through to see the city in a variety of artificial hues. To your right is the former Farmers and Mechanics Savings Bank of Minneapolis, now the posh Westin Hotel. The front of the building is decorated with a large relief sculpture of a farmer and mechanic in Art Deco style, while the interior of the hotel has retained the original 1940s walnut paneling.

If you're any sort of history buff at all, you may want to dawdle a bit in the Wells Fargo Center, home of the somewhat-hagiographic Wells Fargo History Museum. After looking at the displays, the exit into the next skyway is ahead of you and to the left.

- Go straight through the skyway. This takes you to Gaviidae Common, a small but upscale shopping mall originally designed by César Pelli in the 1980s. A gorgeous bronze loon statue serves as a fountain with a two-story drop into a blue-tiled pool below, while the ceiling is a sky-blue arch broken up by skylights.

Minneapolis City Hall from downtown skyway

- Turn left at the end of the walkway and right at the information booth to enter the skyway. You are now in the City Center building. Turn left past the escalator to get to the next skyway and into the Macy's building.

- Follow the left walkway through Macy's and take the first strong left to get to the skyway leading to the IDS Center.

  The IDS Center is a good place to get a feel for local culture. Downstairs, you'll find the Crystal Court, an indoor park with tables and park benches surrounded by bonsai trees decorated year-round in Christmas lights. If you're looking for Minnesota souvenirs to send distant friends and family, Love From Minnesota carries everything from birch-bark knickknacks and Amish-made goods to locally raised honey, syrups, and, of course, wild rice.

- Go past the escalators and enter the skyway into the Baker Center. Follow the path to the left through the building and stay to the left. Go up the incline and into the skyway to the Northstar Center.

- Go through the skyway to the end of the hall and follow the path to the left. Go straight and up the stairs, past Amy's Classic Confections and out the skyway doors.

- Go through the skyway and turn right. Continue straight and up the stairs, and turn right at the end of the hall and into the skyway.

- Go through the U.S. Bank Plaza, turn left, and pass the shoeshine stand to enter the next skyway.

- Take the skyway to the CenturyLink Building, turn left, and follow the walkway past Classic Cookie into the next skyway entrance.

- Go through the Midland Building and into the next skyway.

- Go through the TriTech Office Center and follow the path to the left to get to the next skyway.

- Go through the Towle Building and turn right at the fork to the next skyway.

● Take the skyway to The Crossings building, turn right, and keep to the left to the next skyway.

● Take the Washington Ave. skyway through to the 100 Washington Square building and turn left. Follow the walkway and go out the door at the first exit sign. If you pass the sign, you will eventually end up at a locked condo-complex door and have to back-track, so pay close attention here.

● Go down the stairs and turn right, and then turn left. Go past the Downtown Market and out the door to the street.

POINTS OF INTEREST

Tea House ourteahouse.com, 330 2nd Ave. S., Towle Building, Minneapolis, MN 55401, 612-343-2133

Classic Cookie mplsclassiccookie.mysite.com, 200 5th St. S., #295, Wells Fargo Midland Building, Minneapolis, MN 55402, 612-338-1949

Amy's Classic Confections skywaymyway.com, 601 Marquette Ave., Northstar Center, Minneapolis, MN 55402, 612-436-0016

Wells Fargo History Museum wellsfargohistory.com, 90 7th St. S., Wells Fargo Building, Minneapolis, MN 55402, 612-667-4210

Gaviidae Common gaviidaecommon.com, 651 Nicollet Mall, Minneapolis, MN 55402, 612-372-1230

City Center tinyurl.com/mncitycenter, 33 6th St. S., Minneapolis, MN 55402

IDS Center ids-center.com, 80 8th St. S., Minneapolis, MN 55402

Love From Minnesota lovefrommn.com, 80 8th St. S., #178, IDS Center, Minneapolis, MN 55401, 612-333-2371

route summary

1. Enter the Churchill building, go past Downtown Market, and take the first left. Go upstairs and turn right into the skyway.

2. Enter The Crossings building and go straight. Turn left at the elevators into the skyway.

3. Enter the Towle Building, go straight, and turn left. Go out the doors and into the skyway.

4. Go straight through the TriTech Building, out the doors to your right, and into the Wells Fargo Midland Building. Follow the path past the escalator and go straight to the skyway.

5. Follow the walkway through the U.S. Bank Plaza to the skyway.

6. Enter the Canadian Pacific Plaza building, go straight past the escalators, and turn right. Go downstairs, go straight, and make a left at the end of the hall into the skyway.

7. Enter Northstar Center, go straight, and turn right at Amy's Classic Confections to enter the skyway.

8. Go straight through the Wells Fargo building to enter the skyway.

9. Go straight through Gaviidae Common and turn left at the end of the walkway to enter the skyway.

10. Go straight through the City Center building and turn left at the escalator to enter the skyway.

11. Follow the left path through Macy's and take your first hard left to enter the skyway.

12. Enter IDS Center and turn right. Enter the skyway to go to the Baker Center.

13. Enter Northstar Center, go up the stairs, go straight past Amy's Classic Confections, and go out the skyway doors.

14. Go through the skyway and turn right. Go straight and up the stairs, and turn right at the end of the hall and into the skyway.

15. Go through the U.S. Bank Plaza, turn left, and go straight past the shoeshine stand to enter the next skyway.

16. Go through the Wells Fargo Midland Building and into the next skyway.

17. Take the skyway to the CenturyLink Building, turn left, and follow the walkway past Classic Cookie to enter the skyway.

18. Go through the TriTech Office Center and follow the left path to enter the skyway.

19. Go through the Towle Building and turn right at the end of the walkway.

20. Take the skyway to The Crossings building, go straight, and make a left. Follow the walkway to the next skyway.

21. Enter the Churchill building, follow the walkway, and go out through the first exit sign.

22. Go down the stairs, turn left, and turn left again. Go past the Downtown Market and out the door to the street.

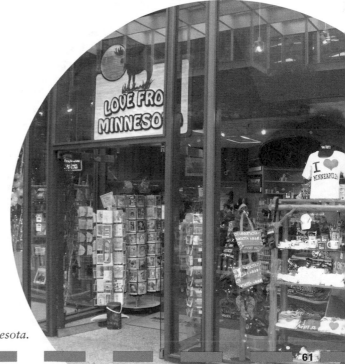

Find souvenirs galore at Love From Minnesota.

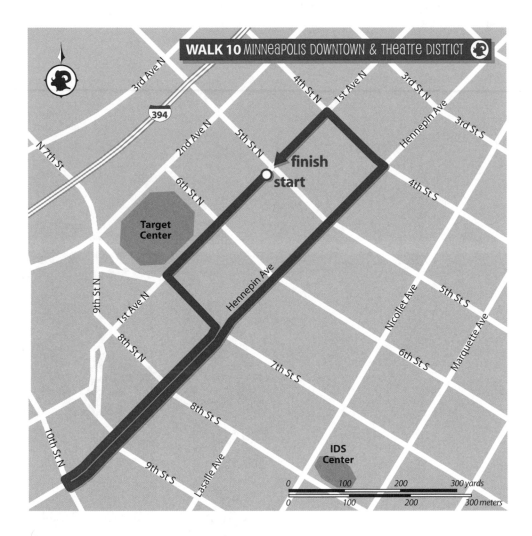

finish
start

394

Target
Center

IDS
Center

3rd Ave N

N 7th St

2nd Ave N

5th St N

6th St N

4th St N

1st Ave N

3rd St N

Hennepin Ave

3rd St S

4th St S

9th St N

1st Ave N

8th St N

Hennepin Ave

7th St S

Nicolet Ave

5th St S

6th St S

Marquette Ave

10th St N

8th St S

9th St S

LaSalle Ave

0   100   200   300 yards
0   100   200   300 meters

10 MINNEAPOLIS DOWNTOWN & THEATRE DISTRICT: SHOWS & DRINKS

BOUNDARIES: **10 St. N., 1st Ave. N., 4th St. N., Hennepin Ave.**
HUDSON'S TWIN CITY STREET ATLAS **COORDINATES:** **Map 394, 2B**
DISTANCE: **Approx. 1 mile**
DIFFICULTY: **Easy**
PARKING: **Limited street parking and parking ramps on 1st Ave. N. or 5th St. N.**
PUBLIC TRANSIT: **Bus lines 7, 14, and 94**

The Twin Cities is second only to New York City in live theater performances and attendance per capita, and nowhere is this more apparent than in the Theatre District in downtown Minneapolis. Since the 1920s, the Orpheum, State, and Pantages Theatres have opened their stages to the likes of the Marx brothers, Jack Benny, George Burns and Gracie Allen, and, more recently, live productions of *The Lion King*—which premiered at the Orpheum—and *The Graduate*, starring Kathleen Turner. All three venues also offer great live music and comedy, with touring acts as varied as Margaret Cho, Eric Idle, Bebel Gilberto, and Modest Mouse. This walk takes you through this historic neighborhood, as well as all the cool places to hang out before and after theater events.

● **Start at 1st Ave. N. and 5th St. N. The light-rail train goes down 5th St. to the station to your left from here. Pick up a route schedule at the station for future use.**

● **Cross 5th St. N. to follow 1st Ave. N. On your left is a charming mural that spans the side of the fantastic Gluek's Restaurant & Bar—in operation since 1933, it's the oldest restaurant in downtown Minneapolis. Aside from their small but wonderful trans-fat-free menu, this is the best place to buy a mug of rich and creamy Gluek's beer.**

● **Cross 7th St. N. Directly in front of you is the star-covered First Avenue nightclub, which has brought in acts as diverse as Iggy Pop, Ice-T, and Stereolab for more than 30 years. You may recognize First Avenue from scenes in Prince's film *Purple Rain*, and if not, you'll probably recognize many of the club's past performers, whose names are spray-painted on the stars covering the building.**

- Turn left to follow 7th St. N. and walk alongside First Avenue nightclub. The small door leading into the side of the building is the club's smaller "subclub"—the 7th Street Entry, which brings many international touring bands to a more intimate setting and also features good local bands just starting out. Right next door to 7th Street Entry is First Avenue's newest addition, the Depot Tavern.

- Turn right on Hennepin Ave. On your right is the Pantages Theatre. The recently relocated Brave New Workshop is a comedy institution founded by Dudley Riggs, a former Ringling Bros. and Barnum & Bailey aerialist who created the organization's precursor, the Instant Theatre in New York City. After touring with that group, he moved to Minneapolis in the 1950s and changed the name. Fifty-plus years after it was founded, it continues its mission with comedy shows, stand-up, and improv. The Saloon and the former Amsterdam Hotel upstairs are some of the last remnants from the area's notorious past of prostitution and clandestine, pre-Stonewall gay bars. The Saloon is famous for mixing some of the strongest drinks in town. Next door is the Orpheum Theatre.

- Take a left at 10th St. N. to cross Hennepin Ave. The giant church on your left is the First Baptist Church, built in 1885.

- Take an immediate left to go back up Hennepin on the other side of the street.

- Cross 9th St. N. This takes you right past the beautiful State Theatre. The Skyway Show Lounge—now Lure Showclub—is the last remaining strip club on the block, and it is also where the author of *Candy Girl* and *Juno,* Diablo Cody, worked briefly as a stripper.

- Cross 7th St. N. On the left side of the street is the former Hennepin Center for the Arts, now a part of the Cowles Center for Dance and the Performing Arts, located inside a gigantic former Masonic temple built in 1889. Within the building's eight floors reside more than 17 performing and visual art companies. Next door is the historic Shubert Theatre.

- Cross 5th St. N. To your right is the massive Lumber Exchange Building. Built in 1885, it's the oldest building taller than 12 stories outside of New York City and the first building to be billed as fireproof in the country. On the left side of the street is Gay

90's, the largest gay and lesbian entertainment complex in the upper Midwest, with eight bars, two restaurants, a drag lounge, male strip show, leather-only bar, and three huge dance floors. It also has a bingo night.

- Turn left onto 4th St. N. Cross Hennepin and go straight to the corner of 1st Ave. N. and 4th St. N.

- Turn left to go to 5th St. N., the starting point.

POINTS OF INTEREST

Gluek's Restaurant & Bar glueks.com, 16 6th St. N., Minneapolis, MN 55403, 612-338-6621

First Avenue and 7th Street Entry/The Depot Tavern first-avenue.com, 701 1st Ave. N., Minneapolis, MN 55403, 612-332-1775

Pantages Theatre hennepintheatretrust.org/our-theatres/pantages-theatre, 710 Hennepin Ave., Minneapolis, MN 55403, 612-373-5600

Brave New Workshop theatre.bravenewworkshop.com, 824 Hennepin Ave., Minneapolis, MN 55401, 612-332-6620

The Saloon saloonmn.com, 830 Hennepin Ave., Minneapolis, MN 55403, 612-288-0459

Orpheum Theatre hennepintheatretrust.org/our-theatres/orpheum-theatre, 910 Hennepin Ave., Minneapolis, MN 55403, 612-339-7007

First Baptist Church fbcminneapolis.org, 1021 Hennepin Ave., Minneapolis, MN 55403, 612-332-3651

State Theatre hennepintheatretrust.org/our-theatres/state-theatre, 805 Hennepin Ave., Minneapolis, MN 55403, 612-339-7007

Lure Showclub lurempls.com/the-club, 725 Hennepin Ave., Minneapolis, MN 55403, 612-886-1056

Cowles Center for Dance and the Performing Arts thecowlescenter.org, 528 Hennepin Ave., Minneapolis, MN 55403, 612-206-3636

Gay 90's gay90s.com, 408 Hennepin Ave., Minneapolis, MN 55401, 612-333-7755

route summary

1. Start at 1st Ave. N. and 5th St. N.

2. Cross 5th St. N. to follow 1st Ave. N.

3. Cross 7th St. N. and turn left.

4. Turn right on Hennepin Ave.

5. Turn left at 10th St. N. and take an immediate left to return on Hennepin in the opposite direction.

6. Turn left on 4th St. N.

7. Turn left at 1st Ave. N. and 4th St. N. and go straight to the corner of 1st Ave. N. and 5th St. N., the starting point.

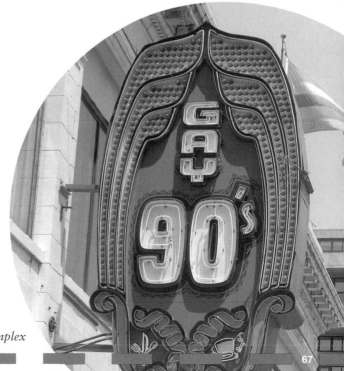

Gay 90's entertainment complex

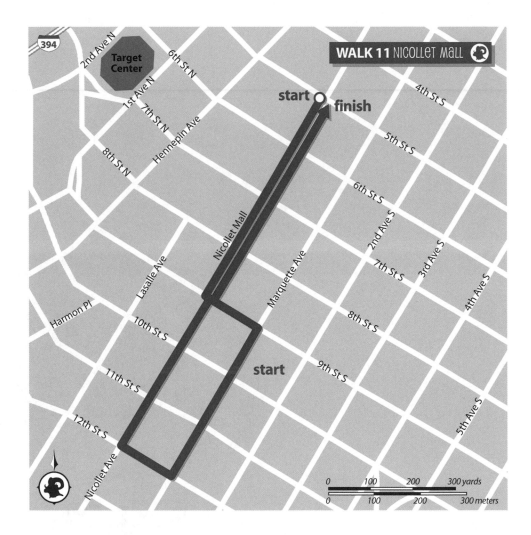

394

2nd Ave N

Target Center

6th St N

1st Ave N

7th St N

8th St N

Hennepin Ave

start

finish

4th St S

5th St S

6th St S

Nicollet Mall

Lasalle Ave

Marquette Ave

2nd Ave S

7th St S

3rd Ave S

Harmon Pl

10th St S

8th St S

4th Ave S

11th St S

start

9th St S

12th St S

5th Ave S

Nicollet Ave

0   100   200   300 yards

0   100   200   300 meters

11 NICOLLET MALL: ART, CULTURE, & MARY TYLER MOORE

BOUNDARIES: **12th St. S., Nicollet Mall, 5th St. S., Marquette Ave.**
HUDSON'S TWIN CITY STREET ATLAS COORDINATES: **Map 394, 2B and 2C**
DISTANCE: **Approx. 1¼ miles**
DIFFICULTY: **Easy**
PARKING: **Metered parking on 5th St. S. and Nicollet Mall, with parking ramps nearby**
PUBLIC TRANSIT: **5th St. light-rail station stop one block from starting point; bus lines 10, 11, 17, 18, and 25**

Located in the heart of downtown Minneapolis, Nicollet Mall is 12 blocks of flower-lined sidewalks with ample opportunities for window-shopping, closed off to all street traffic except for bicycles, taxis, and city buses. This section of Nicollet Avenue was converted into one of the country's first pedestrian malls in 1967, laid out in a gentle S-shape that was later revisited as a C-curve in 1987 to accommodate new construction. On select days from late November until just before Christmas, the mall is home to the famous Holidazzle Parade, an electric parade that makes its way down the tree-lined streets. Every Thursday May–October, one of the oldest and most popular urban farmers' markets is held here, and the streets are packed with local merchants selling everything from fresh fruit to handmade musical instruments.

● Start at the southeast corner of 5th St. S. and Nicollet Mall. Cross 5th St. S. to follow Nicollet Mall. You'll also find a kiosk right here with maps and information about the neighborhood. At 555 Nicollet Mall is the street entrance to Gaviidae Common.

● Cross 7th St. S., continuing southwest. This takes you past the gigantic triangular sculpture that marks the street-level entrance to the IDS Center's Crystal Court.

● Cross 8th St. S. and go straight. You'll see the massive downtown Barnes & Noble, which is a great place to buy a cup of hot chocolate (and a book) before braving the cold to watch the Holidazzle Parade. Next door at 801 Nicollet Mall is the McGladrey Plaza building, which was the fictional home of WJM-TV, the TV station where Mary Tyler Moore worked in the show bearing her name (although most of the episodes were actually filmed in Los Angeles). On the corner is Zelo, which serves wonderful Italian food and desserts in an elegant setting.

● Cross 9th St. S. and take a left. This takes you by the Young-Quinlan Building at 81 9th St. S., named after Elizabeth Quinlan, the first and only woman clothing buyer in the U.S. when her ready-to-wear store opened in 1894. The building, ornamented with extraordinary scrollwork and elegant details, stands as a lavish centerpiece of Minneapolis's high-end shopping district. It's also the only public building in Minneapolis that still uses human elevator operators. Haskell's founder, Benny Haskell, was a liquor provider to the area well before the store's official opening in 1934—Haskell was a bootlegger during the days of Prohibition, delivering his goods from a Cadillac touring car with drawn side curtains.

● Turn right at the corner of Marquette Ave. and 9th St. S. to follow Marquette Ave. From here, you can see the full scope of the Foshay Tower at 821 Marquette Ave. Completed in 1929 just months before the Great Depression, it remained the tallest structure in Minneapolis until 1972, when the neighboring IDS Center was built. It's still the second-highest concrete skyscraper in the country, right after the Empire State Building. In the Handicraft Guild Building, you'll find Dahl Violin Shop, a high-end violin shop opened in the 1920s by Mathias Dahl, who claimed to have received the formula for his special wood varnish directly from the spirit of Antonio Stradivari. On the far corner to your right is the back side and garden of local TV station WCCO.

● Cross 11th St. S. and go straight, continuing southwest. This takes you past Orchestra Hall, home of the Minnesota Orchestra and an amazing place to catch classical and jazz music acts from around the world.

● Turn right at 12th St. S. and go straight. Across the street is the massive stone Westminster Presbyterian Church, built in 1896. The church, which features a gigantic, 16-foot-wide stained glass rose window, provides daily tours. To the right is Peavey Plaza, where you can hear live music most afternoons throughout the summer in a garden setting next to a cooling fountain. The Twin Cities Jazz Festival is also held here, and events from Orchestra Hall often spill over into the plaza.

- Cross the street at Nicollet Mall and turn right to follow Nicollet Mall. This takes you by Brit's Pub, a popular English-themed pub, as well as the high-end French restaurant Vincent A Restaurant, both located in the ornate Lafayette Building.

- Cross 11th St. S. and continue straight, heading northeast. Across the street is the front side of the WCCO TV station, where you can watch the news as it's being reported through the big glass windows in front. To your left is the upscale Mexican restaurant Masa, which serves contemporary Mexican cuisine with an emphasis on seafood dishes. Just down the street, the Dakota Restaurant & Jazz Club is both the best place in town to catch live jazz music and possibly the best restaurant in the Twin Cities for American cuisine.

- Cross 10th St. S. and go straight. On the right side of the street is the Local Irish Pub, which is actually three small bars in one: the Victorian-style Porter Pub, a dark room furnished with big stuffed armchairs and sofas around a fireplace; the well-lit and lunch-friendly Willy Reilly's; and the self-explanatory Whiskey Lounge, with more than 300 whiskey bottles on display. This part of the walk also takes you past the ornate storefront façade of the Young-Quinlan Building and the beautiful Elliot Offner sculpture, *Three Bird Fountain,* which depicts three Minnesotan birds: the great blue heron, the loon, and the sage grouse. On the corner of 7th St. S. stands a bronze statue of Mary Tyler Moore throwing her hat into the air, in the exact spot that she did in the opening credits of *The Mary Tyler Moore Show.*

- Go straight until you cross 5th St. S. to finish the walk.

POINTS OF INTEREST

Gaviidae Common gaviidaecommon.com, 651 Nicollet Mall, Minneapolis, MN 55402, 612-372-1230

IDS Center ids-center.com, 80 8th St. S., Minneapolis, MN 55402

Barnes & Noble bn.com, 801 Nicollet Mall, Minneapolis, MN 55402, 612-371-4443

Zelo zelomn.com, 831 Nicollet Mall, Minneapolis, MN 55402, 612-333-7000

Haskell's haskells.com, 81 9th St. S., Minneapolis, MN 55402, 800-486-2434

Dahl Violin Shop 89 10th St. S., Ste. 205, Minneapolis, MN 55403, 612-339-4800

Orchestra Hall minnesotaorchestra.org, 1111 Nicollet Ave., Minneapolis, MN 55403, 612-371-5600

Westminster Presbyterian Church ewestminster.org, 1200 Marquette Ave., Minneapolis, MN 55403, 612-332-3421

Brit's Pub britspub.com, 1110 Nicollet Mall, Minneapolis, MN 55403, 612-332-3908

Vincent A Restaurant vincentarestaurant.com, 1100 Nicollet Mall, Minneapolis, MN 55403, 612-630-1189

Masa masa-restaurant.com, 1070 Nicollet Mall, Minneapolis, MN 612-338-6272

Dakota Restaurant & Jazz Club dakotacooks.com, 1010 Nicollet Ave., Minneapolis, MN 55414, 612-332-1010

Local Irish Pub the-local.com, 931 Nicollet Mall, Minneapolis, MN 55402, 612-904-1000

route summary

1. Start at the corner of 5th St. S. and Nicollet Mall, on the southwest side of the street.
2. Go straight to follow Nicollet Mall until you get to 9th St. S.
3. Cross 9th St. S., and turn left.
4. Turn right onto Marquette Ave. and go straight.
5. Turn right at 12th St. S. and go straight.
6. Turn right on Nicollet Ave. and turn right again to follow Nicollet Mall.
7. Go straight until you get to 5th St. S. to finish the walk.

The IDS Center, built in 1972

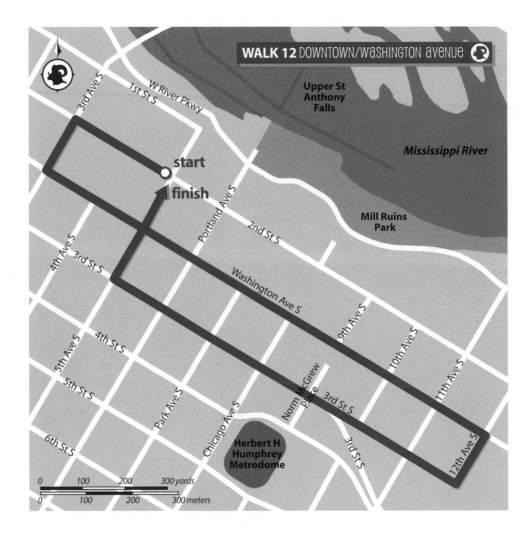

Upper St
Anthony
Falls

Mississippi River

Mill Ruins
Park

3rd Ave S

1st St S

W River Pkwy

start

finish

Portland Ave S

2nd St S

4th Ave S

3rd St S

Washington Ave S

9th Ave S

10th Ave S

11th Ave S

5th Ave S

4th St S

5th St S

Park Ave S

Chicago Ave S

Norm McGrew
Place

3rd St S

3rd St S

12th Ave S

6th St S

Herbert H
Humphrey
Metrodome

| 0 | 100 | 200 | 300 yards |
| 0 | 100 | 200 | 300 meters |

12 DOWNTOWN/WASHINGTON AVENUE: A NEW FOCUS FOR AN OLD NEIGHBORHOOD

BOUNDARIES: **3rd St. S., 3rd Ave. S., 2nd St. S., 12th Ave. S.**
HUDSON'S TWIN CITY STREET ATLAS **COORDINATES:** **Map 394, 3B**
DISTANCE: **Approx. 1¾ miles**
DIFFICULTY: **Easy**
PARKING: **Metered parking on 2nd St. S.**
PUBLIC TRANSIT: **Bus line 7**

The Downtown neighborhood, just off the Mill District, is another area in flux. Less than 20 years ago, it mostly consisted of abandoned warehouse buildings, machine shops, and lots of parking ramps, with the big white bubble of the Metrodome as the key point of interest.

Today, this neighborhood is home to one of the largest literary collectives in the country and a world-renowned theater, as well as upscale restaurants, publishing houses, and architectural firms. A walk down Washington Avenue means a stroll among old railroad beds converted into parking lots, as well as candy factories and meatpacking plants converted into performance spaces for National Endowment for the Arts prizewinning poets and writers.

● **Start on the corner of 5th Ave. S. and 2nd St. S. with the MacPhail Center for Music at your back. Walk past the Residence Inn by Marriott, formerly the Milwaukee Road Depot—built in 1899 and in use until 1971. Now, the spacious building comprises not only a hotel but also a great indoor water park open to nonhotel guests for a fee. Even though locals still fume that the more glamorous Union Depot, formerly located near the Hennepin Avenue Bridge, wasn't preserved as well, it's still nice that this lovely old building, with its attached clock tower and ornate boarding platform, has been saved from the wrecking ball. Ahead and to your right is the Carlyle Condos building, the tallest residential building in Minneapolis.**

● **Turn left at 2nd St. S. and 3rd Ave. S. On the corner is Dunn Bros.' Freight House, located in the original freight house serving the Milwaukee Road Depot. This Dunn Bros. sells great coffee drinks and pastries and also regularly hosts live music. On** the right side of the street at 220 Washington Ave. S. is the United States Federal Office Building, which briefly served as the city's main post office.

- Turn left at Washington Ave. S. to head southeast. Continue straight, past the depot and its elegant, covered boarding platform, which now serves as a parking lot for hotel guests.

- Cross 5th Ave. S. On your left is Colombian figural artist Fernando Botero's bronze sculpture of two portly nudes dancing.

  Cross the street at Portland Ave. S., and continue walking on the other side of Washington Ave. S.

- Cross Park Ave. S. and continue southeast. On the left side of the street, the renovated old lumber, textile, and flour mill ruins—now glitzy condos—provide a wonderful glimpse of the area's past and present. The building with the big star on top is the former North Star Woolen Mill, while the Washburn A Mill and Ceresota Flour buildings have retained the original faded logos painted on their sides. The building with the giant crater on top is the Mill City Museum (see Walk 15). To your right is the big white bubble of the Hubert H. Humphrey Metrodome, where the Vikings play football—soon to be replaced by a state-of-the-art stadium slated to open in 2016. To the left is the blue curve of the Guthrie Theater, a bastion of Twin Cities' live theater since 1963, and at this particular location since 2006.

  The big brick building at 1011 Washington Ave. S. is the Open Book building, which houses the largest literary collective in the country. Inside is the Minnesota Center for the Book Arts, which offers classes on bookmaking; the Loft Literary Center, a creative writing school for adults and children; and the Coffee Gallery, which sells soups, sandwiches, coffee, and pastries. Big Brain Comics is a comic book store for serious comic book readers. It carries all the Marvel and DC superhero fare but is mostly known for its selection of manga and graphic novel selections. Grumpy's is a great bar and restaurant owned by former Halo of Flies front man and Amphetamine Reptile Records owner, Tom Hazelmyer.

- Turn right at 12th Ave S. Go straight and turn right at the STOP sign to follow 3rd St. S.

- Cross 10th Ave. S. and cut through the parking lot, angling to the left. This takes you to the squat and angular building that's home to the free baseball museum Dome Souvenirs Plus, founded by Ray Crump, former batboy for the Washington Senators and the Twins' first equipment manager. Right across the street is the Metrodome, home of the Minnesota Twins baseball team until late 2009.

- Cross Norm McGraw Place/9th Ave. S. and go straight. Ahead is downtown Minneapolis. To the right, you can see most of the old Mill District on either side of the river, as well as the Guthrie Theater. Ahead and to the left, you can see the big arched roof of the Minneapolis Armory, where the Minnesota Lakers played basketball before moving to Los Angeles in the 1960s.

- Cross 5th Ave. S., and then turn right to follow it.

- Cross Washington Ave. S. and go straight. On the right, the MacPhail Center for Music is a school for young musicians. The school holds regular lunchtime concerts that are free and open to the public—an easy thing to appreciate, even if you don't have kids attending the school. Up ahead is 2nd St. S. and 5th Ave. S., our starting point.

POINTS OF INTEREST

Freight House/Dunn Bros. Coffee freighthouse.dunnbros.com, 201 3rd Ave. S., Minneapolis, MN 55401, 612-692-8530

Mill City Museum millcitymuseum.org, 704 2nd St. S., Minneapolis, MN 55401, 612-341-7555

Hubert H. Humphrey Metrodome msfc.com, 900 5th Ave. S., Minneapolis, MN 55415, 612-332-0386

Guthrie Theater guthrietheater.org, 818 2nd St. S., Minneapolis, MN 55415, 612-377-2224

Open Book openbookmn.org, 1011 Washington Ave. S., Ste. 100, Minneapolis, MN 55415, 612-215-2520

Big Brain Comics bigbraincomics.com, 1027 Washington Ave. S., Minneapolis, MN 55415, 612-338-4390

Grumpy's grumpys-bar.com/downtown, 1111 Washington Ave. S., Minneapolis, MN 55415, 612-340-9738

Dome Souvenirs Plus domeplus.com, 910 3rd St. S., Minneapolis, MN 55415, 612-375-9707

MacPhail Center for Music macphail.org, 501 2nd St. S., Minneapolis, MN 55401, 612-321-0100

route summary

1. Start on the corner of 5th Ave. S. and 2nd St. S.
2. Go down 2nd St. S., and turn left at 3rd Ave. S.
3. Turn left at Washington Ave. S.
4. Turn right at Portland Ave. S. to cross Washington Ave.
5. Turn left to walk down the other side of Washington Ave. S.
6. Turn right at 12th Ave. S.
7. Turn right at 3rd St. S.
8. Cross 10th Ave. S. and cut through the parking lot, angling to the left.
9. Cross Norm McGraw Place/9th Ave. S. and go straight.
10. Cross 5th Ave. S. and turn right to follow 5th Ave. S. until 2nd St. S. to finish the walk.

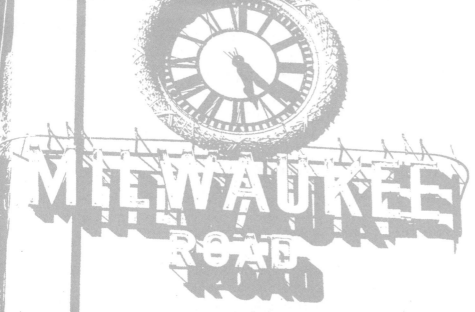

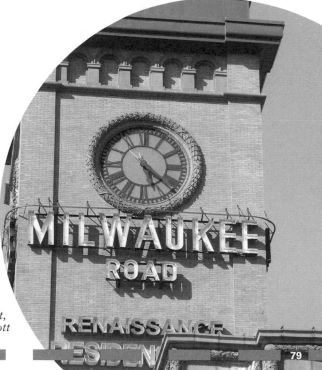

Milwaukee Road Depot,
now a Residence Inn by Marriott

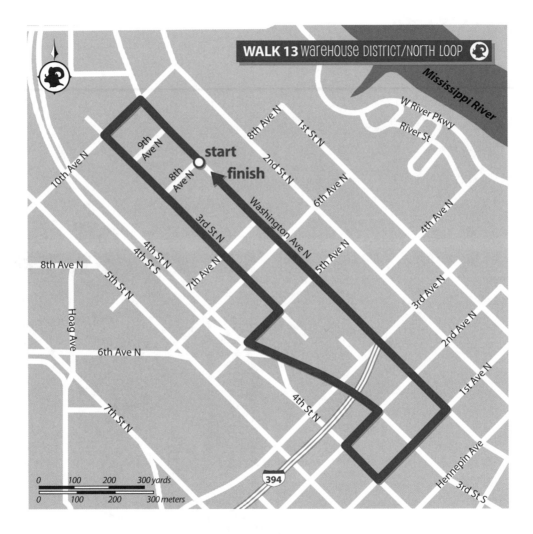

WALK 13 Warehouse District/North Loop

Mississippi River

W River Pkwy

River St

8th Ave N

1st St N

2nd St N

6th Ave N

9th Ave N

8th Ave N

start
finish

10th Ave N

Washington Ave N

4th Ave N

3rd St N

5th Ave N

3rd Ave N

8th Ave N

4th St N

4th St S

7th Ave N

2nd Ave N

5th St N

Hoag Ave

6th Ave N

1st Ave N

4th St N

7th St N

Hennepin Ave

3rd St S

0   100   200   300 yards
0   100   200   300 meters

394

13 Warehouse District/North Loop: The Oldest "New" Neighborhood

BOUNDARIES: 1st Ave. N., 4th St. N., 10th Ave. N., Washington Ave. N.
HUDSON'S TWIN CITY STREET ATLAS **COORDINATES:** Map 394, 2B
DISTANCE: Approx. 2 miles
DIFFICULTY: Moderate
PARKING: Metered parking on Washington Ave.
PUBLIC TRANSIT: Bus line 14

With the completion of the transcontinental railroad systems in the 1860s, Minneapolis became an important wholesale trade center for the country. By the early 1920s, more than 300 warehouse businesses, including paper, paint, and farm machinery manufacturers, were located here in Minneapolis, and with these new businesses came lots of money. Some of the greatest architects of the day were hired to design these buildings, and they did so with flair.

The North Loop neighborhood of Minneapolis's Warehouse District features an amazingly intact concentration of late-19th- to early-20th-century commercial buildings, spared from the wrecking ball not from any appreciation of the architecture but simply because the city couldn't afford to demolish the buildings. Today, these buildings have been converted into remarkable condos, restaurants, and nightclubs. No doubt the new Twins baseball stadium will also influence the area's development.

- **Start at the TractorWorks Building (800–828 Washington Ave. N.), built in 1902. The building, decorated with a large high relief stag head over the entrance, served as the Minneapolis headquarters for the farm-implement company John Deere. This is where you'll find Be'Wiched Deli, which makes amazing sandwiches on a variety of homemade breads, using local, natural, and sustainable food sources.**

- **Go straight to follow Washington Ave. northeast.**

- **Cross 10th Ave. N. and turn left to follow 10th Ave. N. southwest.**

- Turn left at 3rd St. N. and go straight, heading southeast. Some of the better condo developments in recent years are here at 918 Lofts (918 3rd St. N.) and Bassett Creek Lofts (901 3rd St. N.).

- Cross 8th Ave. N. and continue southeast. On the corner you'll find the fenced-in North Loop Dog Grounds. On the right side of the street (701 3rd St. N.) is the ornate Sherwin-Williams Company's former Minneapolis headquarters building. Throughout this area you'll notice hints of the huge paper-milling district once here, including the C. J. Duffey Paper Company, Litin Paper Company, Falk Paper Company, and the *Star Tribune* newspaper's paper-manufacturing building.

- Cross 6th Ave. N. and go straight. Across the street (525 3rd St. N.) is the Bookmen Loft Condo building—originally the Bookmen Printing Building. On this side of the street is Corner Coffee, which serves up live acoustic music with its great coffee and food, for lunch and for late-night crowds, Monday–Saturday.

- At 5th Ave. N., cross the street. Then turn right and go straight to continue to follow 5th Ave. N.

- Just after the STOP sign at 4th St. N., turn left to take the sidewalk that goes under the I-94 on-ramp. (If you're thirsty, turn right, following the underpass sidewalk, and turn left on 6th Ave. On your right, a half block away, you'll see the Fulton Brewery Tap Room.) Off to your right is the Twins baseball stadium, Target Field, completed in 2010. Below you are both defunct and working train tracks and a light-rail stop for the stadium, while to your left is a great panoramic view of the Warehouse District.

- Follow the path down to 2nd Ave. N. and cross the street. Turn right to head south-west on 2nd Ave. N.

- Turn left at 4th St. N. Across the street is the historic Textile Building, built in 1891, where you'll find local favorite restaurant Pizza Lucé. At the corner and on the right side is the spectacularly ornate Wyman Building at 400 1st Ave. N., built in 1896. Until recently, the Wyman Building was occupied by local artists and private gallery owners, but due to the rising rental costs, the building is now mostly occupied by architectural firms, real estate investors, and upscale bars.

● Turn left at 1st Ave. N. On your left is the gray stone hulk of the **Consortium Building**, built in 1887. At 241 1st Ave. N. is the **Lerner Publishing Group**, a successful publisher of children's books that has resided at this address since 1959.

● Turn left at Washington Ave. N. **One on One Bicycle Studio** is a live-music venue and art gallery that serves coffee drinks and even runs a bicycle repair shop in the back. The gigantic brick building near the corner houses **Sex World** and its side club, **Sinners**. Open 24 hours a day, Sex World is one of the largest sex shops in the country, with several floors of live entertainment, including cage dancers and glass-fronted peep shows, with several more floors dedicated to selling merchandise and displaying erotic art from local and national artists. Sex World had one of the first Internet coffee shops in the city, though the coffee itself is of pretty poor quality.

● Cross the iron railroad bridge and continue northwest. You're now in the middle of the Warehouse District/North Loop neighborhood—and in a fabulous picture-taking spot. On the right, the **Free Spirit building** (428 Washington Ave. N.) is home to Free Spirit Publishing, another award-winning publisher of children's books. On the left is **Gardner Hardware**—in operation at this site since 1884, it's one of the last of the independent hardware stores in the region. On the right is **Black Sheep**, an East Coast–style, coal-fired pizzeria. On your left is **Smack Shack**, home of all things lobster. Its trademark lobster roll sandwich was named one of the best in the country by *Bon Appétit* magazine—not bad, considering that Minneapolis is well over a thousand miles away from any lobster traps. On the right is the **International Harvester Company of America building** (618 Washington Ave. N.), built in 1916 and a former distribution site for farm machinery. It's now the Harvester Lofts, an upscale condo development. At 701 Washington Ave. N. is the former factory building for **Loose-Wiles Biscuit Company**; built in 1910, it features a gorgeously menacing stone lion over the entranceway.

● Cross 8th Ave. N. Across the street is the **TractorWorks Building**, where you'll finish the walk.

POINTS OF INTEREST

Be'Wiched Deli bewicheddeli.com, 800 Washington Ave. N., Minneapolis, MN 55401, 612-767-4330

North Loop Dog Grounds doggrounds.org, 3rd St. N. and 8th Ave. N., Minneapolis, MN 55401

Corner Coffee yourcornercoffee.com, 514 3rd St. N., #102, Minneapolis, MN 612-338-2002

Fulton Brewery Tap Room fultonbeer.com, 414 6th Ave. N., Minneapolis, MN 55401, 612-333-3208

Target Field minnesota.twins.mlb.com/min/ballpark, 1 Twins Way, Minneapolis, MN 55403, 612-338-9467

Pizza Lucé pizzaluce.com, 119 4th St. N., Minneapolis, MN 55401, 612-333-7359

One on One Bicycle Studio oneononebike.com, 117 Washington Ave. N., Minneapolis, MN 55401, 612-371-9565

Sex World/Sinners shopsexworld.com, 241 2nd Ave. N., Minneapolis, MN 55401, 612-672-0556

Gardner Hardware Co. gardnerhardwareco.com, 515 Washington Ave. N., Minneapolis, MN 55401, 612-333-3393

Black Sheep blacksheeppizza.com, 600 Washington Ave. N., Minneapolis, MN 55401, 612-342-2625

Smack Shack smack-shack.com, 603 Washington Avenue N., Minneapolis, MN 55401, 612-379-4322

ROUTE SUMMARY

1. Start at the TractorWorks Building at 800–828 Washington Ave. N. Go northwest along Washington Ave.
2. Turn left at 10th Ave. N. and go straight, heading southwest.
3. Turn left at 3rd St. N. and go straight, heading southeast.
4. At 5th Ave. N., cross the street, turn right, and go straight southwest.
5. Just after the STOP sign at 4th St. N., turn left to take the sidewalk under the I-94 on-ramp.
6. Cross 2nd Ave. N. and turn right to follow 2nd Ave. N.

7.   Turn left at 4th St. N. and go southeast.

8.   Turn left at 1st Ave. N. and go straight, heading northeast.

9.   Turn left at Washington Ave. N. Go straight (northwest) to 8th Ave. N. to finish the walk.

Downtown Minneapolis

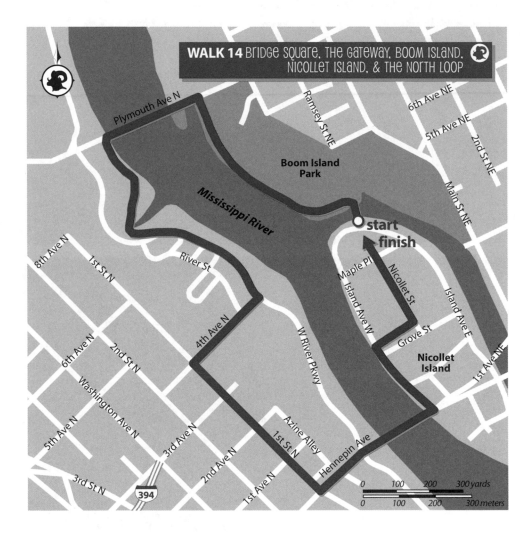

WALK 14 BRIDGE SQUARE, THE GATEWAY, BOOM ISLAND, NICOLLET ISLAND, & THE NORTH LOOP

Plymouth Ave N

Ramsey St NE

6th Ave NE

5th Ave NE

2nd St NE

Boom Island Park

Mississippi River

Main St NE

start
finish

8th Ave N

1st St N

River St

Maple Pl

Nicollet St

Island Ave E

6th Ave N

2nd St N

4th Ave N

Island Ave W

Grove St

Nicollet Island

1st Ave NE

Washington Ave N

5th Ave N

3rd Ave N

W River Pkwy

2nd Ave N

Azine Alley

1st St N

Hennepin Ave

3rd St N

1st Ave N

| 0 | 100 | 200 | 300 yards |
| 0 | 100 | 200 | 300 meters |

394

14 Bridge Square, The Gateway, Boom Island, Nicollet Island, & The North Loop: Old Town Reinvented

BOUNDARIES: 1st St. N., Plymouth Ave. N., Main St. N.E., Nicollet St., Hennepin Ave. E.
HUDSON'S TWIN CITY STREET ATLAS **COORDINATES:** Map 394, 2A, 3A, 2B, and 3B
DISTANCE: Approx. 2 miles
DIFFICULTY: Easy
PARKING: Free 4-hour parking on Island Ave. E. and Island Ave. W.
PUBLIC TRANSIT: Bus line 11

Minneapolis was born on the shores of the then-murky Mississippi River. Bridge Square and the Gateway District were the original housing and government centers of the hardworking city in the 19th century. In the early years of the Mill City, lumbering was the main source of wealth, and Boom Island was where the branded logs were sorted. The Gateway was then the locus of the city, where Hennepin Ave. and Nicollet Ave. converged, with Bridge Square at the south side of the Hennepin Avenue Bridge. Nicollet Island remained a blighted industrial area until the 1960s, and Basset Creek in the 1850s was the site for at least seven sawmills. Until the 1950s, the area was an industrial warehouse district. In the past few decades, the area has been transformed. First came the arts organizations, restaurants, nightclubs, and coffee shops. Then came the renovated and newly constructed condos, lofts, and townhomes to form the residential North Loop that we see today. Nicollet Island is now a place where nature and beautifully restored Victorian homes exist within walking distance from downtown, while the Gateway and Bridge Square areas have long since been incorporated into downtown's business and residential district.

● Begin on Nicollet Island, at the top of the steps where Island Ave. E. and Island Ave. W. converge. Descend the railroad-tie stairs, turn left, and cross the pedestrian bridge to Boom Island. The iron truss bridge was salvaged from the Wisconsin Central Railroads—an industrial advancement that made the island a misnomer because the eastern channel is now connected to the mainland.

- Turn left at the fork, and at the next two pedestrian intersections, follow the path closest and parallel to the Mississippi River.

- Turn left at the *Minneapolis Queen* and the *Paradise Lady* boat launch area. The two riverboats offer public cruises on the Mississippi River, passing through the Minneapolis Riverfront District.

- Follow the pedestrian bridge across the channel leading to the steps of the Plymouth Avenue Bridge.

- Turn left at the top of the stairs on the Plymouth Avenue Bridge. The bridge provides a scenic vista of downtown to the south and of Nordeast on the east side of the river.

- Turn left to go south on W. River Pkwy. and follow the center pedestrian path (stay out of the bicycle lane). Across the parkway is the North End neighborhood.

- Turn left at the Grand Rounds information kiosk and follow the path downhill toward the river, winding through peaceful urban parkland lined with mature trees and plentiful plant species.

- Turn left at the sign for the bridge that crosses Bassett Creek. The creek was named after lumberman Joel Bassett, who in 1852 built a farm and the first steam-powered sawmill in the vicinity. Sadly, for much of the city's history, 1½ miles of the creek have been diverted into a concrete storm sewer under Minneapolis that runs into the Mississippi River. Additional rustic walking paths are available for exploration of the creek and its surroundings.

- Turn left at the end of the bridge, stay on the middle cement sidewalk along the river, and then go immediately left again.

- After passing the parking lot on W. River Pkwy., turn right on 4th Ave. N. to go southwest. Here you'll see a couple of huge condo projects—the gated Landings on the right and Renaissance on the River on the left.

- Turn left on 1st St. N. On the right are a number of striking condo renovations and constructions, such as the Rock Island Lofts.

- Continue and cross the bridge. On the left is Bachelor Farmer, owned by Governor Mark Dayton's sons, which serves gourmet comfort food with a Scandinavian twist. If you're not careful, you'll walk right past this wonderful, understated restaurant's front door without noticing it. In the summer, Bachelor Farmer holds its annual *kräftskiva,* featuring a crawfish boil and local beer and music. A block ahead and on the right is the Alliance Française, an organization that promotes French culture through language classes, lectures, social events, music, and film at various sites throughout the Twin Cities.

- Continue forward, crossing 1st Ave. N. On the left is Origami Restaurant. The restaurant features excellent sushi as well as a selection of the best sakes, wines, scotches, beers, and mixed drinks.

- Turn left on Hennepin Ave., where the Federal Reserve Bank—once the locus of Bridge Square—is located. Kitty-corner from the intersection of 1st Ave. N. and Hennepin Ave. is the George Washington Memorial Flagstaff (1917)—the only object that remains, although slightly moved, from the original Gateway Park and the Gateway District.

- Continue on the Hennepin Avenue Bridge. Italian horror director Dario Argento shot his first American film, *Trauma*, in Minneapolis in 1993. It's on this bridge that the director's daughter, Asia, attempts suicide in the movie—with the local landmark, the Grain Belt Beer sign, behind her.

- At the end of the bridge, make an immediate left, descend the stairs, and turn right at the bottom of the stairs. On the right is DeLaSalle High School, a Catholic high school on the island since 1900.

View from Boom Island

THE GATEWAY DISTRICT & BRIDGE SQUARE: THE OTHER OLD TOWN MINNEAPOLIS

During the early years of Minneapolis, Bridge Square and the neighboring Gateway District were central to the development of the nascent city. Bridge Square was the area located immediately across the Hennepin Avenue Bridge, and adjacent was the Gateway, where Nicollet Ave. and Hennepin Ave. converged to form the hub of the developing city. In 1850 Colonel John Stevens built a home—long since relocated to Minnehaha Park—on a site near the current U.S. Post Office building, where Minneapolis and Hennepin County were founded. Here the first of the four bridges spanning the east and west banks of the Mississippi was built in 1855. Goose Pond was contained in Bridge Square early in its history. The pond's location diverted traffic in the direction of the present route of Nicollet Mall, toward Fort Snelling. Shortly after the pond was drained in 1882, a 275-foot-high light tower was constructed to illuminate the city, only to be torn down after 10 years due to system failures. Later, the city developed massive projects such as the Great Northern Railroad (1914) and Gateway Park Pavilion (1915) that replaced the original small buildings.

This was the beginning of a long, dramatic end for Bridge Square. The Gateway District became the working-class center of the city, with hundreds of flophouses and bars for the transient population. Eventually the area became a skid row and the pavilion a sad and decaying hobo hangout. In 1957 the city began its downtown revitalization when 17 blocks were leveled. Gateway Park Pavilion was one of numerous historic buildings, some dating back to the 1850s, demolished. The area's significance declined in the vastly expanding city—the Gateway Park was replaced by enormous uninspired condos, apartments, and office buildings. Bridge Square is now occupied by busy thoroughfares and the Federal Reserve Bank (1997).

- Continue straight across Grove St. To the right are the Eastman Flats (1877), an excellent example of French Second Empire row houses constructed with lovely local limestone.

- Continue forward, crossing the railroad tracks. At the park's parking lot, turn right and follow the path through the woods.

- Turn left on Nicollet St. and take in the beautiful Victorian homes.

- Continue straight on Nicollet St. until it ends, and then follow the paved path through the park and woods to finish the walk.

POINTS OF INTEREST

Boom Island Park tinyurl.com/boomisland, 724 Sibley St. N.E., Minneapolis, MN 55413, 612-230-6400

Minneapolis Queen **and** *Paradise Lady* twincitiescruises.com, Plymouth Ave. and Boom Island Park, Minneapolis, MN 55413, 612-378-7966

The Bachelor Farmer thebachelorfarmer.com, 50 North 2nd Ave., Minneapolis, MN 55401, 612-206-3920

Alliance Française afmsp.org, 113 1st St. N., Minneapolis, MN 55401, 612-332-0436

Origami Restaurant origamirestaurant.com, 30 1st St. N., Minneapolis, MN 55401, 612-333-8430

Nicollet Island Park tinyurl.com/nicollet, 724 Sibley St. N.E., Minneapolis, MN 55413, 612-230-6400

route summary

1. Begin at the top of the steps on Nicollet Island where Island Ave. E. and Island Ave. W. converge. Go down the railroad-tie stairs, turn left, and cross the pedestrian bridge to Boom Island.

2. Turn left at the fork, and at the next two pedestrian intersections, follow the path closest and parallel to the Mississippi River.

3. Turn left at the *Minneapolis Queen* and *Paradise Lady* boat launch area.

4. Follow the pedestrian bridge across the channel leading to the steps to the Plymouth Avenue Bridge.

5. Turn left at the top of the stairs on the Plymouth Avenue Bridge.

6. Turn left on W. River Pkwy. and follow the center pedestrian path.

7. Turn left at the Grand Rounds information kiosk, and follow the path downhill toward the river as it winds through the park.

8. Turn left at the bridge sign.

9. Turn left at the end of the bridge, stay on the middle cement sidewalk along the river, and then immediately go left again.

10. Turn right on 4th Ave. N. after passing the parking lot on W. River Pkwy.

11. Turn left on 1st St. N.

12. Continue and cross the bridge.

13. Continue forward, crossing 1st Ave. N.

14. Turn left on Hennepin Ave.

15. Continue on the Hennepin Avenue Bridge.

16. At the end of the bridge, make an immediate left, go down the stairs, and turn right at the bottom of the stairs.

17. Continue straight across Grove St.

18. Continue forward, crossing the railroad tracks. At the park's parking lot, turn right and follow the path through the woods.

19. Turn left on Nicollet St.

20. Continue straight on Nicollet St. until it ends, and then follow the paved path through the park and woods to finish the walk.

Crayfish from the Bachelor Farmer kräftskiva

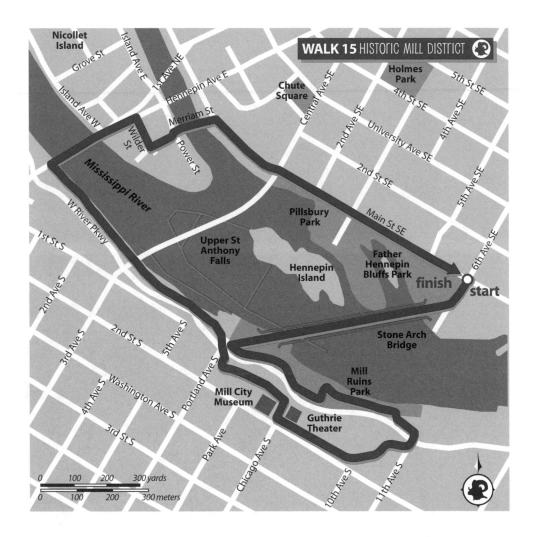

Nicollet
Island

Grove St

Island Ave E

1st Ave NE

Hennepin Ave E

Chute
Square

Central Ave SE

2nd Ave SE

University Ave SE

Holmes
Park

4th St SE

5th St SE

4th Ave SE

Island Ave W

Merriam St

Wilder
St

Power St

2nd St SE

5th Ave SE

Mississippi River

Pillsbury
Park

Main St SE

W River Pkwy

Upper St
Anthony
Falls

Hennepin
Island

Father
Hennepin
Bluffs Park

1st St S

2nd Ave S

2nd St S

5th Ave S

6th Ave SE

finish

start

Stone Arch
Bridge

3rd Ave S

Washington Ave S

4th Ave S

Portland Ave S

Mill City
Museum

Mill
Ruins
Park

3rd St S

Park Ave

Chicago Ave S

Guthrie
Theater

10th Ave S

11th Ave S

0   100   200   300 yards
0   100   200   300 meters

15 HISTOrIC MILL DISTrICT: INDUSTrIAL WASTELAND reNewed as scenic urban playground

BOUNDARIES: 6th Ave. S.E., 11th Ave. S., W. River Pkwy., 2nd St. S., Hennepin Ave. E., Main St. S.E.
HUDSON'S TWIN CITY STREET ATLAS **COORDINATES: Map 394, 3B**
DISTANCE: Approx. 2½ miles
DIFFICULTY: Moderate
PARKING: Limited free parking on 2nd St. and 6th Ave.; metered parking on Main St.
PUBLIC TRANSIT: Bus lines 7, 17, and 22

The Historic Mill District is not a neighborhood but a confluence of historic Minneapolis communities surrounding the city's quintessential life source: waterpower from St. Anthony Falls. Energy was a limited commodity in the 19th century, and the abundant hydroelectric source provided an accessible, affordable, and consistent supply. As a result, industry—followed by communities—developed on both east and west banks of the energy-rich Mississippi River.

The city of St. Anthony, on the east bank, came into existence in 1838 under the leadership of lumber and milling entrepreneur Franklin Steele. Minneapolis, on the west bank, was not founded until 1852 but flourished after annexing St. Anthony in 1872. The proximity to waterpower and the farms of the Upper Midwest transformed Minneapolis into a world leader in flour production 1880–1920. In this milieu, two giants in the industry—General Mills and Pillsbury—emerged and consolidated the industry, later becoming omnipresent, diversified national brands. However, the milling industry gradually decentralized, and General Mills moved its headquarters to suburban Golden Valley and closed the Washburn A Mill in 1965. The descent began, and the area was largely abandoned until the 1970s. The renovation began in Old St. Anthony, reaching a crescendo with the condo building boom at the beginning of the new century. The industrial birthplace of Minneapolis has become one the city's most beautiful locales—a fact that would, no doubt, amaze those early pioneers.

● **Start at the corner of 6th Ave. S.E. and Main St. S.E., and follow the sidewalk south toward the Stone Arch Bridge. On the right is Father Hennepin Bluffs Park, where in**

1680 the captive Belgian Louis Hennepin was the first European to encounter St. Anthony Falls, named in honor of Hennepin's patron saint—St. Anthony of Padua.

- Turn right to cross the Stone Arch Bridge. The bridge was constructed in 1883 by James J. Hill to complete his St. Paul, Minneapolis, and Manitoba Railroad, which later became the Great Northern Railroad. The only stone bridge on the Mississippi, the immense limestone bridge cuts diagonally across the river for 2,100 feet. It remained in operation until 1978 and reopened after renovation as a pedestrian and bicycle bridge in 1994.

- At the end of the bridge, immediately turn left and enter Mill Ruins Park, where you can catch a glimpse of the remains of first-generation mills along the river.

To your right are examples of Minneapolis's longtime ties with waterpower. Starting in 1857, the Minneapolis Mill Company, a consortium, controlled and operated the water-power on the west side of the river with 25 flour mills and 30 industrial buildings. In 1885 the consortium deepened and lengthened the canal to use as its power source.

- Continue descending on the path and turn right. On the left are the Upper St. Anthony Falls Lock and Dam, with an observation area and public restroom.

- Turn right and follow the metal staircase across the tailrace. Here, you can read about the area's history and archeology dig findings, documented on markers.

- Turn left on the metal boardwalk after exploring the mill ruins.

- At the end of the sidewalk, turn right and go uphill toward the enormous mills and the intersection of 11th Ave. and W. River Pkwy., passing the I-35W Bridge Remembrance Garden.

- After crossing W. River Pkwy., follow the middle path through Gold Medal Park. The park was named after the General Mills flour of the same name, which won the Miller's Exhibition in Cincinnati in 1880 and brought national prominence to the brand.

- Turn right on 2nd St. S., passing the park's large sign. From here, you can see the Guthrie Theater and the Mill City Museum, with downtown in the background.

- Continue northwest, toward architect Jean Nouvel's internationally acclaimed Guthrie Theater (2006). The French architect designed the theater with this site in mind, and it fits in well beside the immense renovated mills. Not only does it include three theaters, but it also has a restaurant, bars, and a cantilever overhanging W. River Pkwy.

- Turn right at the huge picture of Sir Tyrone Guthrie on the side of the theater. On the left is Spoonriver Restaurant, owned by local culinary legend Brenda Langton. At Spoonriver, she has added organic and grass-fed meats to the delicious menu, which includes weekend brunches. In the shed between the restaurant, the Mill City Museum, and the Guthrie is the Mill City Farmers Market, held on Saturday, May–October.

- Turn left. On the left is the Washburn A Mill Complex (1880), home of the company that, through mergers, became General Mills. The first Washburn A Mill exploded on May 2, 1878, killing 18 in one of the city's greatest industrial disasters. The second A Mill was vacant for a number of years and caught fire in 1991, destroying much of the roof and walls. In 2003, the ruins were renovated and redesigned by Meyer, Scherer & Rockcastle, Ltd. as a multiuse structure that includes the Mill City Museum, restaurants, and condos. The museum, operated by the Minnesota Historical Society, features exhibits and an elevator ride to a rooftop observation deck.

- Turn right at the MILL RUINS PARK sign, crossing W. River Pkwy., and turn left on the pedestrian path. On Saturdays in the summer, kids age 8 and older can join ongoing archeological digs here (preregistration is required).

- Turn right, following the riverside pedestrian path, and turn left next to the waterpower headrace. On the left

Mill Ruins Park

is a series of historic mills, such as the Crown Roller Mill (1878), which was renovated and converted into office space.

● Continue northwest under the 3rd Avenue Bridge. Up ahead is the U.S. Post Office (1934), an enormous three-block Art Deco Mankato Kasota Stone building. Well worth a visit is First Bridge Park, located directly ahead. Here you can stop to read the interpretive information on the four bridges that have occupied the site since it became the first permanent span across the Mississippi River in 1855.

● Turn left to go up the first set of stairs, and turn right onto the Hennepin Avenue Bridge.

● Turn right on Wilder St. The Nicollet Island Pavilion and park for St. Anthony Falls is straight ahead—a detour to this scenic spot is well worth it.

● Turn left after crossing Merriam St. and continue along it. On the left is the Nicollet Island Inn, a swanky destination for fine dining, five-course meals, and Sunday brunches, plus elegant lodging in the converted Island Sash and Door Works (1893). Until the middle of the 20th century, Nicollet Island was a vast industrial area packed with factories and not the pristine park you see today.

● After crossing the Merriam Street Bridge, turn right on Main St. S.E. The bridge was salvaged from the Broadway Avenue Bridge upriver to become one of the four spans. On the left is Riverplace, developed in 1984 as a mall and restaurant complex—unfortunately, only restaurants remain in this former urban mall. The Wilde Roast Cafe serves gourmet comfort food and award-winning desserts in an intimate setting. After passing under the 3rd Avenue Bridge you'll see St. Anthony Main Theatre on the left, where the Minneapolis–St. Paul International Film Festival is held every spring. Next door is Pracna (1890), a restaurant and bar with elegant food and specialty beers. It's also where the rebirth of Old St. Anthony began—Pracna was used first as a residence in 1969, then converted into a restaurant a few years later. At the end of the block is the Aster Café (1855), a relaxing place to enjoy coffee, sandwiches, soups, and salads in Minneapolis's oldest extant commercial building. Tuggs Tavern offers reasonably priced drinks and bar food with free live music in the courtyard during the summer. On the right is the most recent addition to Old St. Anthony—Water Power Park, where walkers are afforded a view above St. Anthony Falls.

● Cross 3rd Ave. S.E. The enormous, historic Pillsbury A Mill, with limestone walls 8 feet thick in some areas, is presently in the controversial process of being converted into condos. On the right are stairs leading down to Hennepin Island via the Lower Path—a beautiful piece of nature where you can get a good, close look at the crumbling brick façades of old factories. Unfortunately, erosion has resulted in the closure of sections of the already-rough trail.

● Finish the walk at the intersection of Main St. S.E. and 6th Ave. S.E.

POINTS OF INTEREST

Father Hennepin Bluffs Park/Stone Arch Bridge tinyurl.com/hennepinbluffs, 420 Main St. S.E., Minneapolis, MN 55414, 612-230-6400

Mill Ruins Park tinyurl.com/millruins, 103 Portland Ave. S., Minneapolis, MN 55401, 612-230-6400

Upper St. Anthony Falls Lock and Dam nps.gov/miss/planyourvisit/uppestan.htm, 1 Portland Ave. S., Minneapolis, MN 55401, 612-333-5336

Gold Medal Park nps.gov/miss/planyourvisit/goldmedal.htm, 2nd St. S. and 11th Ave. S., Minneapolis, MN 55415, 612-230-6400

Guthrie Theater guthrietheater.org, 818 2nd St. S., Minneapolis, MN 55415, 612-377-2224

Spoonriver Restaurant spoonriver.com, 750 2nd St. S., Minneapolis, MN 55401, 612-436-2236

Mill City Museum millcitymuseum.org, 704 2nd St. S., Minneapolis, MN 55401, 612-341-7555

Mill City Farmers Market millcityfarmersmarket.org, 704 2nd St. S., Minneapolis, MN 55401, 612-341-7580

First Bridge Park tinyurl.com/firstbridgepark, 1 W. River Pkwy., Minneapolis, MN 55401, 612-230-6400

Nicollet Island Park tinyurl.com/nicollet, 724 Sibley St. N.E., Minneapolis, MN 55413, 612-230-6400

St. Anthony Park tinyurl.com/stanthonypark, Jefferson St. N.E. and Spring St. N.E., Minneapolis, MN 55413, 612-230-6400

Nicollet Island Inn nicolletislandinn.com, 95 Merriam St., Minneapolis, MN 55401, 612-331-1800

Wilde Roast Cafe wilderoastcafe.com, 65 Main St. S.E., Minneapolis, MN 55414, 612-331-4544

St. Anthony Main Theatre stanthonymaintheatre.com, 115 Main St. S.E., Minneapolis, MN 55414, 612-331-4723

Pracna pracnaminneapolis.com, 117 Main St. S.E., Minneapolis, MN 55414, 612-379-3200

Aster Café aster-cafe.com, 121 Main St. S.E., Minneapolis, MN 55414, 612-379-3138

Tuggs Tavern tuggstavern.com, 219 Main St. S.E., Minneapolis, MN 55414, 612-379-4404

Water Power Park tinyurl.com/waterpwrpark, 204 Main St. S.E., Minneapolis, MN 55414, 612-230-6400

route summary

1. Start at the corner of 6th Ave. S.E. and Main St. S.E. and follow the sidewalk straight toward the Stone Arch Bridge.

2. Turn right to cross the Stone Arch Bridge.

3. Turn left immediately at the end of the bridge and enter the Mill Ruins Park.

4. Go down the path and turn right.

5. Turn right and follow the metal staircase across the headrace.

6. Turn left on the metal boardwalk.

7. At the end of the sidewalk, turn right and go uphill toward the enormous mills and the intersection of 11th Ave. and W. River Pkwy.

8. After crossing W. River Pkwy., follow the middle path through Gold Medal Park.

9. Turn right on 2nd St. S., passing the park's large sign.

10. Turn right at the huge picture of Sir Tyrone Guthrie on the side of the theater.

11. Turn left on the sidewalk next to the plank road.

12. Turn right, crossing W. River Pkwy. (at the MILL RUINS PARK sign) and turn left on the pedestrian path.

13. Turn right, following the riverside pedestrian path, and left on the pedestrian path next to the waterpower headrace.

14. Continue under the 3rd Avenue Bridge.

15. Turn left, go up the first set of stairs, and turn right on the Hennepin Avenue Bridge.

16. Turn right on Wilder St.

17. Turn left after crossing Merriam St.

18. Cross the Merriam Street Bridge, and turn right on Main St. S.E.

19. Finish the walk at the intersection of Main St. S.E. and 6th Ave. S.E.

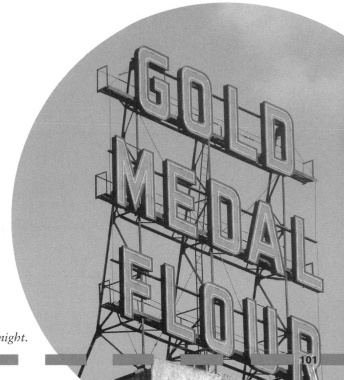

The Gold Medal Flour sign is lit up at night.

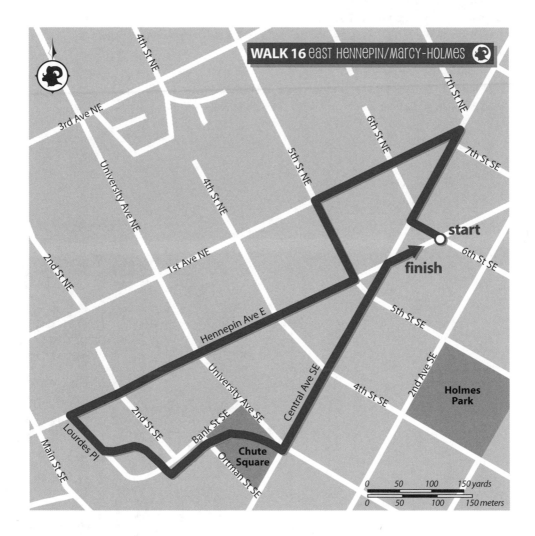

start

finish

Holmes
Park

Chute
Square

4th St NE

3rd Ave NE

University Ave NE

4th St NE

5th St NE

6th St NE

7th St NE

7th St SE

2nd St NE

1st Ave NE

Hennepin Ave E

6th St SE

5th St SE

4th St SE

2nd Ave SE

2nd St SE

University Ave SE

Bank St SE

Central Ave SE

Lourdes Pl

Ortman St SE

Main St SE

0   50   100   150 yards
0   50   100   150 meters

16 east Hennepin/marcy-Holmes: where southeast & northeast meet

BOUNDARIES: Central Ave. S.E., Lourdes Place, Hennepin Ave. E., 1st Ave. N.E., 7th St. N.E.
HUDSON'S TWIN CITY STREET ATLAS COORDINATES: **Map 394, 3A and 3B**
DISTANCE: **Approx. 1¼ miles**
DIFFICULTY: **Easy**
PARKING: **Free parking on 6th St. S.E.**
PUBLIC TRANSIT: **Bus lines 2 and 4**

A little more than a decade ago, you would have been hard-pressed to find anyone truly excited about visiting this little area that weaves in and out of both Northeast and Southeast Minneapolis. Today it's a destination for haute couture shopping and dining. Previously, this mostly dilapidated historic district was where now-defunct shops such as Cashman's Furniture and Bank's department store struggled to bring in customers. These days, however, the area has been reborn into something of an extension of nearby downtown Minneapolis, with all the glamour and sophistication of the uptown district.

● **Start at Hennepin Ave. E. and 6th St. S.E. in front of Brasa Rotisserie.**

● **Carefully cross Hennepin Ave. E., heading northwest, and go straight to the STOP sign by the Holiday gas station. Across the street at 523 Hennepin Ave. E. is the former site of the original Totino's Pizza—that's right, the creators of those thin frozen pizzas and bite-size pizza rolls. After nearly 56 years at this location, the restaurant moved to the cheaper suburbs in 2007, but the trademark mural of the Totino's pizza man is still there on the wall.**

● **Turn right to follow Central Ave. S.E. and go straight (northeast). The Seafood Market carries a wide selection of fresh fish, as well as a few in-house dishes.**

● **Turn left to cross Central Ave. and go southwest on 1st Ave. N.E. Across the street and to the left is the big Bank's building at 615 1st Ave. N.E., which was a Sears-like discount store for many years before being converted into an office building.**

- Cross 6th St. N.E. and go straight. Across the street is the Red Stag Supperclub, with its distinctive statue of a red stag directly above the sign. The Red Stag shares owners with the upscale Café Barbette and Bryant Lake Bowl & Cabaret Theater, and all three restaurants are notable for serving food crafted from sustainable organic farms. To your left are the Melrose Flats, built in the 1890s—once fairly run-down, they've recently been renovated into snazzy-looking businesses and loft condos.

- Turn left on 5th St. N.E. This takes you along the redbrick façade of the Melrose Flats buildings. Stop and look at the two rock-and-steel Zoran Mojsilov sculptures along the front of Gardens of Salonica, an elegant Greek restaurant open for lunch and dinner, and Melrose Antiques, which sells antiques in mint condition (open by appointment only).

- Turn right at Hennepin Ave. E. to cross 5th St. N.E. and go west along Hennepin Ave. Just down the street is the Bulldog N.E., acclaimed by *Esquire* magazine as one of the best bars in America for the great quality and selection of the food. Across the street to your left is the former site of the Third Northwestern National Bank, now an empty parking lot. On December 16, 1932, one of the bloodiest bank robberies in Minnesota history took place here. The Barker-Karpis gang—linked to Ma Barker and Alvin "Creepy" Karpis—robbed the bank of more than $12,000, killing two Minneapolis police officers and injuring more in the process.

- Cross University Ave. To your right is Kramarczuk's, a family-run deli and restaurant selling homemade sausages, breads, pastries, and other Eastern European cuisine since 1954. Kramarczuk's also hosts an Easter festival and other seasonal events—all with an Eastern European flavor. Across the street to your left is Punch Neopolitan Pizza, an excellent local chain.

- Cross 2nd St. S.E. and turn left to cross Hennepin Ave. E. Make an immediate right to walk in front of Nye's Polonaise Room, declared by *Esquire* magazine to be *the* best bar in America. Built in a former harness shop and tavern, Nye's features a live piano bar that takes requests; the Ruth Adams Polka Band, which bills itself as "the world's most dangerous polka band"; and great Polish food.

● Turn left at Lourdes Pl. On your left is Our Lady of Lourdes Catholic Church, Minneapolis's oldest church. The front part of the church was erected in 1857 for a Universalist congregation but was later sold to a French Catholic group who added the transept, apse, and bell tower in the 1880s. Across the street is the former site of the Industrial Exposition Hall, where the Republican Convention of 1892 nominated incumbent President Benjamin Harrison for a doomed run against Grover Cleveland.

● Turn left to follow the brick sidewalk around Our Lady of Lourdes and make an immediate right. Follow the brick path to the corner and cross Bank St. S.E.

● Turn left. Go straight (northeast).

● Cross Ortman St. S.E. and take a right to follow the path through Chute Square. To your right is the little yellow Ard Godfrey House, the oldest existing wood-frame house in Minneapolis. Built in 1848, the house was moved several times before Chute Square became its permanent location. Ard Godfrey's wife, Harriet, is credited for having brought the first dandelions to Minnesota, and so the Women's Club of Minneapolis holds a Dandelion Days festival every summer in her honor.

● Cross Central Ave. S.E. and turn left to cross University Ave. S.E., walking on Central Ave. On the corner is the former S.E. Library building, now offices for the Phillips Distilling Company. The little building at 326 Central Ave. S.E. was once Jim's Coffee Shop & Bakery, which was featured in the Christian Slater movie *Untamed Heart*. The amazing building that houses the Aveda Day Spa Institute on the corner of Central Ave. S.E. and 4th St. S.E. is the former Cataract Temple, the first Masonic lodge in Minneapolis.

● Turn right to walk northeast along Hennepin Ave. E. Up ahead is Brasa Rotisserie, owned by Alex Roberts (winner of the James Beard Award for Best Chef in the Midwest), on the corner of 6th St. S.E. and Hennepin Ave. E., where we started. Be sure to stop in at Brasa and try some of its wonderful food, which includes rotisserie chicken and pork shoulder roast, all of which is organically raised on local farms.

POINTS OF INTEREST

Brasa Rotisserie brasa.us, 600 Hennepin Ave. E., Minneapolis, MN 55414, 612-379-3030

Seafood Market seafoodmarketmn.com, 628 Central Ave. S.E., Minneapolis, MN 55414, 612-379-6387

Red Stag Supperclub redstagsupperclub.com, 509 6th St. N.E., Minneapolis, MN 55413, 612-767-7766

Gardens of Salonica gardensofsalonica.com, 19 5th St. N.E., Minneapolis, MN 55413, 612-378-0611

Melrose Antiques etsy.com/shop/melroseantiques, 13 5th St. N.E., Minneapolis, MN 55413, 612-362-8480

The Bulldog N.E. thebulldognortheast.com, 401 Hennepin Ave. E., Minneapolis, MN 55414, 612-378-2855

Kramarczuk's kramarczuk.com, 215 Hennepin Ave. E., Minneapolis, MN 55414, 612-379-3018

Punch Neopolitan Pizza punchpizza.com, 210 Hennepin Ave. E., Minneapolis, MN 55414, 612-623-8114

Nye's Polonaise Room nyespolonaise.com, 112 Hennepin Ave. E., Minneapolis, MN 55414, 612-379-2021

Our Lady of Lourdes Catholic Church ourladyoflourdesmn.com, 1 Lourdes Pl., Minneapolis, MN 55414, 612-379-2259

Chute Square tinyurl.com/chutesquare, 28 University Ave. S.E., Minneapolis, MN 55413, 612-230-6400

Ard Godfrey House tinyurl.com/ardgodfrey, 50 University Ave. N.E., Minneapolis, MN 55413, 612-870-8001

Aveda Day Spa Institute avedainstitutemn.com, 400 Central Ave. S.E., Minneapolis, MN 55414, 612-331-1400

route summary

1. Start at Hennepin Ave. E. and 6th St. S.E. in front of Brasa Rotisserie.

2. Carefully cross Hennepin Ave. and go straight up to the STOP sign by the Holiday gas station.

3. Turn right to follow Central Ave. S.E. northeast.

4. Turn left to cross Central Ave. and go southwest on 1st Ave. N.E.

5. Cross 6th St. N.E. and go straight.

6. Turn left on 5th St. N.E.

7. Turn right at Hennepin Ave. E. to cross 5th St. N.E. and go west along Hennepin Ave.

8. Cross 2nd St. S.E. and turn left to cross Hennepin Ave. E. Make an immediate right to walk in front of Nye's Polonaise Room.

9. Make a left at Lourdes Pl.

10. Turn left to follow the brick sidewalk around Our Lady of Lourdes and make an immediate right. Follow the brick path to the corner, and cross Bank St. S.E.

11. Turn left and continue northeast.

12. Cross Ortman St. S.E. and turn right to follow the path through Chute Square.

13. At the corner, cross Central Ave. S.E. and turn left to cross University Ave. S.E. Follow Central Ave.

14. Turn right to follow Hennepin Ave. Up ahead is Brasa Rotisserie on the corner of 6th St. S.E. and Hennepin Ave. E., our starting point.

Kramarczuck's offers Eastern European cuisine.

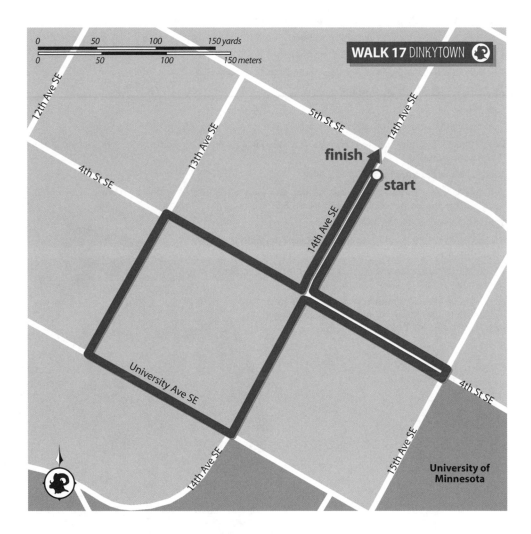

17 DINKYTOWN: THE LITTLE COLLEGE TOWN THAT TRANSCENDS THE GENERATION GAP

BOUNDARIES: **University Ave. S.E., 13th Ave. S.E., 5th St. S.E., 15th Ave. S.E.**
HUDSON'S TWIN CITY STREET ATLAS **COORDINATES: Map 394, 4B**
DISTANCE: Approx. ½ mile
DIFFICULTY: Easy
PARKING: Metered parking on 14th Ave. S.E., 5th St. S.E., and 4th St. S.E.
PUBLIC TRANSIT: Numerous bus lines to Dinkytown

There is a never-ending debate over the origin of the name Dinkytown. The most compelling theories hark back to the small cars for hauling railroad goods and workers, which were called dinkies, or from the long-lost "dinky" movie theater. The approximately five-block commercial district of the Marcy–Holmes neighborhood, nestled just north of the University of Minnesota (U of M) campus, is home to nearly 40 restaurants, numerous live-music venues, and plenty of quirky places to shop. To survive here, businesses must meet the strict tastes of students, college professors, and international students in their search for authenticity, value, and adventure. Dinkytown is the Twin Cities' tiny answer to Greenwich Village.

● Start at the southeast corner of 5th St. S.E. and 14th Ave S.E., and walk southwest. The Subway parking lot was one of the former haunts of Robert Zimmerman, who later changed his name to Bob Dylan. From his freshman year at the U of M in 1959 until he left for quick fame in New York City in 1961, Dylan performed on the window stage at the tiny coffee shop formerly located on this site, the 10 O'Clock Scholar.

● Turn left on the corner of 4th St. S.E. You'll find another excellent recent addition here in Pagoda, a pan-Asian restaurant with an enormous, authentic menu of Chinese regional cuisines—along with Thai, Japanese, Korean, and Malaysian dishes—at reasonable prices.

● Turn right on 15th St. S.E., and then take an immediate right to continue along 4th St. S.E. in the opposite direction. From the railing at the intersection, you get an expansive view of Dinkytown, as well as the distant historic Mill District and downtown

Minneapolis. Just below the railing, you can see that Dinkytown was constructed about a story above the solitary train track below, an area once clogged with rails leading to downtown Minneapolis.

● After crossing 14th Ave., turn left to go southwest. On the right is Loring Pasta Bar, with its stylish and urbane exterior. Glass windows above the entrance are emblazoned with the word *drugs,* a tribute to Gray's Campus Drugs, which occupied this spot for decades before the restaurant and bar opened in 1999. The Loring Bar was a favorite hipster destination in Loring Park until it lost its lease, and owner Jason McLean brought his quirky interior-decorating style to this spot. Just ahead on the right is the Kitty Cat Klub, with the same name as the Berlin nightclub during the interwar period preceding World War II. It is another ultracool spot with drinks, food, and—above all—a hip atmosphere and an outdoor back patio. Next door and upstairs, with another marvelous patio vista, is Annie's Parlour, which has been serving burgers, fries, and malts to several generations of college students.

● Turn right on University Ave. S.E. On the right is the newest location of the Purple Onion Café. The name is a tip-of-the-hat to a coffee shop of the same name during Dylan's brief time in Dinkytown. It moved here after more than a decade at the corner of 4th St. and 14th Ave. and now offers sandwiches, salads, and an expanded menu.

● Turn right on 13th Ave. S.E. Across the street is the Southeast Community Library, formerly the State Capitol Credit Union. The small modernist building was designed in 1964 by U of M architecture professor Ralph Rapson, who died in 2008. On the corner is a "Positively 4th Street" mural, a song that everyone knows was written about Dinkytown and not New York City—at least here, anyway.

● Turn right on 4th St. S.E. On the right is the marquee of the Varsity Theater & Café des Artistes. The old movie theater, long mothballed, was transformed by Jason McLean of the Loring Pasta Bar into one of the area's premier concert venues. The theater is now furnished with couches and other comfy accommodations for lounging with wine or beer and enjoying live music. Across the street is Camdi Restaurant, which serves homey Chinese and Vietnamese food, with plenty of vegetarian and vegan options, at rock-bottom, college-friendly prices.

BOB DYLAN: THE GHOST OF DINKYTOWN

Bob Dylan—known by his birth name, Robert Zimmerman—is a local specter. Dinkytown became his home in 1959 when he arrived from the iron range town of Hibbing, Minnesota, to study at the University of Minnesota. In the company of baby boomers and Dylan fanatics, grand proclamations are made about arguably the greatest songwriter of the modern era. He is the favorite son whose shadow is omnipresent, thanks to the unbelievable success he attained almost immediately after leaving for New York City in January 1961.

The Dinkytown folk scene of this period has a different version of Dylan than the conquering-hero myth that has accrued over ensuing years. Dylan is remembered for being booed off the stage at the tiny 10 O'Clock Scholar during its folk heyday and for purloining rare folk records from contemporaries in the small scene.

Whether Dylan's success was due entirely to talent and ambition or to the desire of his record company, the media, and a growing youth culture to anoint a rough-hewn poet for their generation is debatable. Regardless, Dylan is an international icon who began his career in Dinkytown, and his shadow is cast on everyone and everything in this little neighborhood.

- Turn left on 14th Ave. S.E. This side of the block illustrates the diversity of culinary bounty in Dinkytown. The tiny and legendary restaurant Al's Breakfast serves perfect pancakes, omelets, and eggs Benedict. Just down the block is Kafe 421, fine cuisine at all price ranges, from its student-priced gyros to its superb steaks and bouillabaisse. Finally, next door, Wally's serves good, cheap Middle Eastern food—be sure to try the chicken shawarma.

- Continue northeast on 14th Ave. S.E. to the 5th St. S.E. intersection to finish the walk.

POINTS OF INTEREST

Pagoda pagodadinkytown.com, 1417 4th St. S.E., Minneapolis, MN 55414, 612-378-4710

Loring Pasta Bar loringcafe.com, 327 14th Ave. S.E., Minneapolis, MN 55414, 612-378-4849

Kitty Cat Klub kittycatklub.net, 315 14th Ave. S.E., Minneapolis, MN 55414, 612-331-9800

Annie's Parlour facebook.com/dinkytownannies, 313 14th Ave. S.E., Minneapolis, MN 55414, 612-379-0744

Purple Onion Café thepurpleonioncafe.com, 1301 University Ave. S.E., Minneapolis, MN 55467, 612-252-0217

Southeast Community Library tinyurl.com/secommlibrary, 1222 4th St. S.E., Minneapolis, MN 55414, 612-543-6725

The Varsity Theater & Café des Artistes varsitytheater.org/cafe, 1308 4th St. S.E., Minneapolis, MN 55414, 612-604-0222

Camdi Restaurant camdirestaurant.com, 1325 4th St. S.E., Minneapolis, MN 55414, 612-331-4194

Al's Breakfast 413 14th Ave. S.E., Minneapolis, MN 55414, 612-331-9991

Kafe 421 kafe421.com, 421 14th Ave. S.E., Minneapolis, MN 55414, 612-623-4900

Wally's wallysfalafelandhummus.com, 423 14th Ave. S.E., Minneapolis, MN 55414, 612-746-4776

ROUTE SUMMARY

1. Start at the southeast corner of 5th St. S.E. and 14th Ave. S.E., and walk southwest.
2. Turn left on the corner of 4th St. S.E.
3. Turn right at 15th St. S.E., and then take an immediate right to continue along 4th St. S.E. in the opposite direction.
4. Turn left after crossing 14th Ave. S.E.
5. Turn right on University Ave. S.E.
6. Turn right on 13th Ave. S.E.
7. Turn right on 4th St. S.E.
8. Turn left on 14th Ave. S.E.
9. Continue to the intersection of 14th Ave. S.E. and 5th St. S.E. to finish the walk.

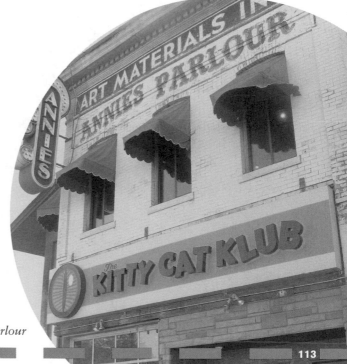

Kitty Cat Klub and Annie's Parlour

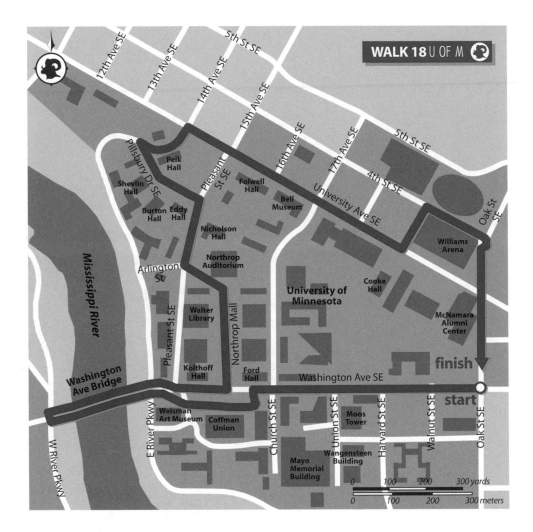

12th Ave SE
13th Ave SE
14th Ave SE
5th St SE
15th Ave SE
16th Ave SE
17th Ave SE
5th St SE
4th St SE
University Ave SE
Oak St SE

Pillsbury Dr SE
Peik Hall
Shevlin Hall
Burton Hall
Eddy Hall
Pleasant St SE
Folwell Hall
Bell Museum
Nicholson Hall
Williams Arena
Arlington St
Northrop Auditorium
Cooke Hall
McNamara Alumni Center

Mississippi River

Pleasant St SE
Walter Library
Northrop Mall
University of Minnesota

Kolthoff Hall
Ford Hall
Washington Ave SE
finish
start
Oak St SE

Washington Ave Bridge
E River Pkwy
Weisman Art Museum
Coffman Union
Church St SE
Union St SE
Moos Tower
Harvard St SE
Walnut St SE

W River Pkwy
Mayo Memorial Building
Wangensteen Building

0   100   200   300 yards
0   100   200   300 meters

18 U OF M: PUBLIC LAND GRANT UNIVERSITY IN THE SHADOW OF DOWNTOWN

BOUNDARIES: **Washington Ave. S.E., W. River Pkwy., 4th St. S.E., Oak St. S.E.**
HUDSON'S TWIN CITY STREET ATLAS COORDINATES: **Map 394, 4B and 4C**
DISTANCE: **Approx. 2½ miles**
DIFFICULTY: **Easy**
PARKING: **2-hour parking on Oak St.; municipal parking lot on the south side of Oak St.**
PUBLIC TRANSIT: **Numerous bus lines to U of M**

The University of Minnesota is the primary postsecondary institution in the state for education and research. Almost everyone in the region has had some contact with the U of M—often simply referred to as The U—as a student or with Golden Gopher sports. The U is a comprehensive public-land-grant university with a national and international reputation in diverse academic disciplines. Esteemed alumni include late journalist Eric Sevareid; Harry Reasoner of television's *60 Minutes*; Garrison Keillor of National Public Radio's *A Prairie Home Companion*; Earl Bakken, inventor of the pacemaker; and Norman Borlaug, the father of the Green Revolution in agriculture. National Baseball Hall of Fame members Dave Winfield and Paul Molitor also attended the U of M, as did Bob Dylan. Another influential dropout was Hubert H. Humphrey, the 1968 Democratic nominee for the U.S. presidency. The architecture, though, is not as outstanding as the school's most successful graduates. Architectural inspiration is often trumped by functionality; still, there are several noteworthy buildings in scenic settings near the Mississippi River. Thrifty and competitive dining options fit the needs of college students in nearby Stadium Village.

● Start at the northwest corner of Oak St. S.E. and Washington Ave. S.E., and walk west on the sidewalk beside the McNamara Alumni Center. Continue through Stadium Village, the small commercial district next to the former location of Memorial Stadium, where the Minnesota Golden Gophers football team played 1924–1981. On the left, after crossing Harvard St. S.E., you'll see the Phillips-Wangensteen Building and Malcolm Moos Health Science Tower—rather uninviting and hulking '70s Brutalist architecture for the world-renowned University of Minnesota medical campus.

- Turn right, following the sidewalk to the base of the bridge, where the path veers left in front of Ford Hall. Turn left to cross the bridge to enjoy the fine view of downtown and the Mississippi River on the right.

- Turn left at the end of the bridge, and then turn right in front of the recently renovated Coffman Union.

- Veer to the right on the sidewalk, passing the reflective stainless steel of the Weisman Art Museum, completed in 1993. It was one of the first art museums designed by Deconstructivist architect Frank Gehry. The University of Minnesota president at the time, Nils Hasselmo, instructed the architect, "Don't build another brick lump." Gehry succeeded by creating a local icon with provocative exterior architecture that has polarized opinions, especially with its trademark geometric shapes and mishmash façade facing the Mississippi River. Inside, the Weisman has many outstanding galleries.

- Turn left on the pedestrian path atop the Washington Avenue Bridge as it crosses the river. From this bridge, poet and U of M English professor John Berryman committed suicide by jumping to his death on a frigid January day in 1972.

- Turn right at the end of the bridge and right again to reverse direction. The West Bank of The U opened in the early 1960s to accommodate the burgeoning student population and has continually expanded. The architecture is functional but relatively uninspiring. The buildings are tied together by a vast network of underground paths. This is a brilliant adaptation, considering the often-inclement weather. It also creates the inaccurate impression aboveground that the area is a ghost town for much of the year.

Below the bridge and slightly upriver on the West Bank is the Bohemian Flats Park, site of the former Bohemian Flats. First settled in the late 19th century, Bohemian Flats had 1,200 residents in the then heavily polluted industrial area in 1900. Until 1963, a few homes still remained in this poor, pan-Slavic immigrant neighborhood. After the tragic collapse of the I-35W Bridge on August 1, 2007, the area served as a salvage area and later as a staging area for the cleanup and reconstruction of the new bridge. Now it's a scenic prairie grass–filled piece of parkland.

- At the end of the bridge, follow the middle pedestrian path above Washington Ave. east toward Northrop Mall. In 1908 local and nationally acclaimed architect Cass Gilbert won a university competition to design future buildings and the mall. Of course, in the battle between artistic vision and economics, the latter won out, and his plan has been severely compromised over the years. The mall did not reach the Mississippi River as planned, and the buildings were constructed of brick rather than stone. The results are functional institutional buildings constructed by architects long after Gilbert had left for larger designs.

- Turn left on the mall at the building on the corner (Kolthoff Hall). On the left, almost at the end of the mall, is the Walter Library, renovated in 2001.

- Walk up the stairs in front of the Northrop Auditorium, and then turn left to go down the stairs as the sidewalk angles right.

- Turn right on Pleasant St. S.E. The street is filled with numerous long-standing campus buildings—some, such as Nicholson Hall, have been renovated within the past decade.

- Turn left on Pillsbury Dr. S.E. On the corner is Eddy Hall. Constructed in 1886 by local architect legend LeRoy Buffington, it's the oldest standing building on campus. Ahead on the left is Burton Hall, another design by Buffington in a Greek Revival style with a Doric portico and columns. Across the street is a bronze sculpture (1900) by Daniel French of U of M regent and Governor John Pillsbury, one of the great early supporters of the fledgling university.

Weisman Art Museum

On the left in front of Shevlin Hall is a stone marking Old Main. Constructed in 1856, it was lost in a 1904 fire. Old Main was the first building at The U after moving from its original location near Chute Square, where it began as a preparatory school in Old St. Anthony.

- Turn right on E. River Pkwy., passing the dull, institutional Peik Hall on the right.

- Turn right on University Ave. S.E., following the wrought iron fence. After crossing Pleasant St. S.E. you'll see on the right the Tudor and Jacobean architecture of Folwell Hall, with its extensive terra-cotta trim around the doors, windows, and roof. The building is named in honor of William Watts Folwell (1869–1884), the school's first president and author of *A History of Minnesota*, a superb four-volume early history of the state.

- Continue southeast on University Ave. S.E. On the left is Chilly Billy's, a locally owned frozen yogurt parlor that stays open extra late for the college crowd. On the right is the Bell Museum of Natural History. It contains dioramas of preserved flora and fauna, as well as hands-on activities for kids. The museum plans to relocate to the St. Paul campus in the indefinite near future. Ahead on the left is the vast majority of the Greek Letter Chapter House Historic District. Between 17th Ave. S.E. and Williams Arena is the greatest concentration of period-revival architecture.

- Turn left at the pedestrian crosswalk before Williams Arena, when you see Cooke Hall on the right. It was from here to Oak St. S.E. that Memorial Stadium once stood and where the Minnesota Golden Gophers won six national championships—unfortunately, they won none after 1960, and they moved to the Hubert H. Humphrey Metrodome in 1982.

- Turn right on 4th St. S.E. and follow the north side of Williams Arena. Since 1928, "the barn" has hosted countless athletic events—most important, home-court games of the Gophers men's basketball team. The classic brown brick exterior is only surpassed by the interior, which still makes for great sports-watching, with its excellent sight lines and lively collegiate atmosphere.

- Continue south, following the contour of Oak St. S.E. as it bends across from the new TCF Bank Stadium.

● Continue following Oak St. S.E. to Washington Ave. S.E. to finish the walk. The colossal copper-covered geode McNamara Alumni Center is at the back of the block and serves as a "front door" to The U. Inside is the Heritage Gallery, honoring the accomplishments of students, alumni, and faculty with the Memorial Stadium Archway as its centerpiece. Across the street is Stub and Herb's Bar and Restaurant, one of the best places in the Twin Cities for Summit, Surly, and Schell's, as well as other local and national microbrews on tap.

POINTS OF INTEREST

McNamara Alumni Center mac-events.org, 200 Oak St. S.E., Minneapolis, MN 55455, 612-624-9831

Stadium Village stadiumvillage.com, University Ave. S.E. and Huron Blvd. S.E., Minneapolis, MN 55455

University of Minnesota umn.edu/twincities, 321 19th Ave. S., Minneapolis, MN 55455, 612-625-2008

Weisman Art Museum weisman.umn.edu, 333 E. River Rd., Minneapolis, MN 55455, 612-625-9494

Bohemian Flats Park tinyurl.com/bohemianflats, 2200 W. River Pkwy., Minneapolis, MN 55406, 612-230-6400

Chilly Billy's chillybillysfrozenyogurt.com, 314 15th Ave. S.E., Minneapolis, MN 55414, 612-843-4278

Bell Museum of Natural History bellmuseum.org, 10 Church St. S.E., Minneapolis, MN 55455, 612-624-7083

Williams Arena umn.edu/twincities, 1925 University Ave. S.E., Minneapolis, MN 55455, 612-624-3514

Stub and Herb's Bar and Restaurant stubandherbsbar.com, 227 Oak St. S.E., Minneapolis, MN 55414, 612-379-1880

route summary

1. Start at the northwest corner of Oak St. S.E. and Washington Ave. S.E., and walk west on the sidewalk beside the McNamara Alumni Center.

2. Turn right as the path veers in front of Ford Hall, and turn left to cross the bridge.

3. Turn left at the end of the bridge, and then turn right in front of Coffman Union.

4. Veer to the right on the sidewalk, passing the reflective stainless steel of the Weisman Art Museum.

5. Turn left on the pedestrian path atop the Washington Avenue Bridge as it crosses the river.

6. Turn right at the end of the bridge and right again to reverse direction.

7. At the end of the bridge, follow the middle pedestrian path above Washington Ave. toward the Northrop Mall.

8. Turn left on the mall at the building on the corner (Kolthoff Hall), following the sidewalk and passing the institutional buildings.

9. Walk up the stairs in front of Northrop Auditorium, and then turn left going down the stairs as the sidewalk angles right.

10. Turn right on Pleasant St. S.E.

11. Turn left on Pillsbury Dr. S.E.

12. Turn right on E. River Pkwy.

13. Turn right on University Ave. S.E., following along the wrought iron fence.

14. Turn left at the pedestrian crosswalk before Williams Arena.

15. Turn right on 4th St. S.E. and follow the north side of Williams Arena.

16. Continue south, following the contour of Oak St. S.E.

17. Continue following Oak St. S.E. to Washington Ave. S.E. to finish the walk.

University of Minnesota, Twin Cities campus

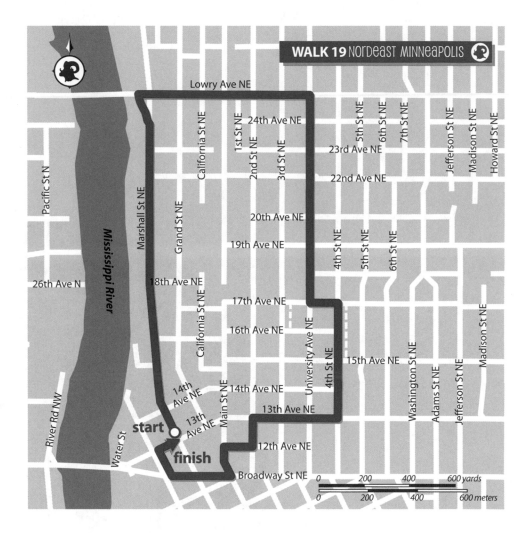

Lowry Ave NE

Pacific St N

Mississippi River

Marshall St NE

California St NE

1st St NE

2nd St NE

3rd St NE

24th Ave NE

23rd Ave NE

22nd Ave NE

5th St NE

6th St NE

7th St NE

Jefferson St NE

Madison St NE

Howard St NE

Grand St NE

20th Ave NE

19th Ave NE

26th Ave N

18th Ave NE

4th St NE

5th St NE

6th St NE

17th Ave NE

16th Ave NE

California St NE

University Ave NE

4th St NE

15th Ave NE

Washington St NE

Adams St NE

Jefferson St NE

Madison St NE

River Rd NW

14th Ave NE

Main St NE

14th Ave NE

13th Ave NE

12th Ave NE

start

13th Ave NE

finish

Water St

Broadway St NE

0   200   400   600 yards
0   200   400   600 meters

19 Nordeast Minneapolis: art, churches, & bars

BOUNDARIES: **Broadway St. N.E., Marshall St. N.E., Lowry Ave. N.E., 4th St. N.E.**
HUDSON'S TWIN CITY STREET ATLAS **COORDINATES: Map 394, 2A and 3A; Map 367, 2D and 3D**
DISTANCE: Approx. 3½ miles
DIFFICULTY: Easy
PARKING: Free 2-hour parking on Marshall St. N.E. and 13th Ave. N.E.
PUBLIC TRANSIT: Bus line 32

For most of Nordeast's history, it was strictly a blue-collar neighborhood, where workers from the nearby Gluek Brewing Company and Minneapolis Brewing Company (later Grain Belt), the rail yards, and the casket and furniture factories made their homes. Many of the original houses were built by the occupants—skilled masons and carpenters—and those few remaining houses attest to their skills.

Since the 1990s, Nordeast has become younger and hipper as artists, writers, and musicians from the Uptown and Warehouse neighborhoods have found themselves priced out of their apartments. Coffee shops, art galleries, and even condos have replaced many of the old neighborhood bars and repair shops; the bars that have managed to stay open through the renaissance have done so by booking local bands and introducing karaoke. Since the mid-1990s, the neighborhood has held the annual Art-a-Whirl gallery tour every May, one of the largest open studio tours in the country—and one more indication that this neighborhood has changed since its early days.

● **Start on the corner of 13th Ave. N.E. and Marshall St. N.E.**

● **Facing Grain Belt Brewery/Pierre Bottineau Community Library, turn right to walk down the left-hand side of Marshall St. N.E.**

● **Follow the sidewalk straight north and across the train tracks. To your left, catch a glimpse of the Mississippi River just past the treeline. The deceptively nondescript** exterior of Psycho Suzi's Motor Lounge hides the fact that there are three tropical-themed tiki bars inside and a riverside patio.

- The tiny Gluek Park reopened in 2007 after undergoing a massive asbestos cleanup. The park gets its name from local beer brewery Gluek (pronounced "glick," in case you want to order one), and you'll see the company's name painted on old warehouse buildings and bars all over town. The Sample Room serves sample plates of cheese, vegetables, and meats, as well as full-size entrées.

- Continue forward, passing the EDGEWATER PARK sign. If you'd like to take a break, follow the path into the park. This isn't the prettiest look at the Mississippi River, but the views from this vantage point—which include a scrap metal recycling center and load-bearing barges passing by—give a good picture of the working-class roots of Minneapolis.

- Turn right at Lowry Ave. N.E..

- Go straight east along Lowry Ave. N.E., all the way to the train tracks. To the right are the downtown Minneapolis skyline, old silos, and warehouse buildings.

- Turn right at University Ave. N.E. Gasthof zur Gemütlichkeit serves a wide selection of tap beers in frighteningly huge boot-shaped glasses. The Gasthof also hosts a popular Oktoberfest party in its parking lot, with German food and live music to accompany the copious quantities of beer served. Downstairs is Mario's Keller Bar, which has live music most nights.

- Cross 22nd Ave. N.E. and continue straight south. The 22nd Avenue Station Bar is the last strip club in the neighborhood and is surrounded almost entirely by churches. On the corner of 20th Ave. N.E. is Jax Café, which is the only restaurant in northeast Minneapolis to feature a trout stream running through the restaurant. For the past 75 years, this has been a favorite dining spot for people of all ages; around prom time you'll find the place packed with young couples in formals. The elegant Kozlak-Radulovich Funeral Chapel at 1918 University Ave. N.E. has been operating here since 1908; it's one of the last reminders that Minneapolis used to be one of the largest coffin producers in the country.

- Cross 17th Ave. N.E. and turn left to cross University Ave. N.E. The Church of the Holy Cross offers a daily Mass in English, and a Sunday Mass in Polish.

- Turn right at 4th St. N.E. and go straight south. Pope John Paul II Catholic School (formerly Church of the Holy Cross Catholic School) is on your right.

- Turn right at the corner at 13th Ave. N.E. Nicholas Harper's Rogue Buddha Gallery—recently relocated here from southeast Minneapolis—is one of the best art galleries in the Twin Cities. The Ritz Theater originally opened in 1928 but was closed for decades before reopening in 2006 as a multimedia event arts venue. S. S. Cyril & Methodius Catholic Church at 1301 2nd St. N.E. features gorgeous stained glass windows and an oxidized copper cupola.

- Cross 2nd St. N.E. and turn left to cross 13th Ave. N.E. Go straight to follow 2nd St. N.E. south. The Frank Stone Gallery is considered the birthplace of the Nordeast gallery scene, in operation here since 1998.

- Turn right at 12th Ave. N.E. The gigantic, ornate building straight ahead is the former Grain Belt Brewery ("the friendly beer with the friendly flavor"), located at Marshall Ave. N.E. and 13th Ave. N.E. The massive, ornately detailed brewery, which was built in 1891, is now home to many local architectural firms, plus a few exclusive galleries.

- Cross Main St. N.E. and take the sidewalk to the left. Turn right to follow west along Broadway St. N.E.

- Cross the street at Marshall St. N.E. This takes you right past the Pierre Bottineau Community Library, established in 2001 and built into the Grain Belt Brewery.

- Cross the tracks and take a right to carefully follow the still-active train tracks. This takes you along the back side of the Grain Belt Brewery building and the nearby former Bottling House, home of local award-winning publisher Coffee House Press. The buildings are made out of yellow brick and echo the lavish Victorian era of their construction.

- Turn right at 13th Ave. N.E. Straight ahead is the corner of Marshall St. N.E. and 13th Ave. N.E., our starting point.

POINTS OF INTEREST

Psycho Suzi's psychosuzis.com, 1900 Marshall Ave. N.E., Minneapolis, MN 55418, 612-788-9069

Gluek Park tinyurl.com/gluek, 2000 Marshall St. N.E., Minneapolis, MN 55418, 612-230-6400

The Sample Room the-sample-room.com, 2124 Marshall St. N.E., Minneapolis, MN 55418, 612-789-0333

Edgewater Park tinyurl.com/edgewaterparkmn, 2326 Marshall St. N.E., Minneapolis, MN 55418, 612-230-6400

Gasthof zur Gemütlichkeit/Mario's Keller Bar gasthofzg.com, 2300 University Ave. N.E., Minneapolis, MN 55418, 612-781-3860

22nd Avenue Station Bar 2121 University Ave. N.E., Minneapolis, MN 55418, 612-789-6793

Jax Café jaxcafe.com, 1928 University Ave. N.E., Minneapolis, MN 55418, 612-789-7297

Church of the Holy Cross ourholycross.org, 1621 University Ave. N.E., Minneapolis, MN 55413, 612-789-7238

Rogue Buddha Gallery roguebuddha.com, 357 13th Ave. N.E., Minneapolis, MN 55413, 612-331-3889

Ritz Theater ritzdolls.com, 345 13th Ave. N.E., Minneapolis, MN 55413, 612-623-7660

S. S. Cyril & Methodius Catholic Church home.catholicweb.com/stcyril, 1315 2nd St. N.E., Minneapolis, MN 55413, 612-379-9736

Frank Stone Gallery frankstonegallery.com, 1224 2nd St. N.E., Minneapolis, MN 55413, 612-617-9965

Pierre Bottineau Community Library hclib.org, 1224 2nd St. N.E., Minneapolis, MN 55413, 612-630-6890

Grain Belt Bottling House and Warehouse artspace.org/our-places/grain-belt-studios, 77 and 79 13th Ave. N.E., Minneapolis, MN 55413, 612-465-0233

route summary

1. Start on the northwest corner of 13th Ave. N.E. and Marshall St. N.E. Walk due north on Marshall St.
2. Follow the sidewalk straight, cross the train tracks, and keep going straight.
3. Turn right at Lowry Ave. N.E.
4. Go straight to follow Lowry Ave. N.E.
5. Turn right at University Ave. N.E.
6. Cross 17th Ave. N.E. and turn left to cross University Ave. N.E.
7. Turn right at 4th St. N.E. and go straight.
8. Turn right at the corner at 13th Ave. N.E.
9. Cross 2nd St. N.E. and turn left to cross 13th Ave. N.E.
10. Turn right at 12th Ave. N.E.
11. Cross Main St. N.E. and take the sidewalk to the left. Turn right to follow Broadway St. N.E.
12. Cross the tracks and take a right to follow the train tracks.
13. Turn right at the street and go straight to the corner of Marshall St. N.E. and 13th Ave. N.E., our starting point.

Historic Grain Belt Brewery building

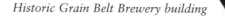

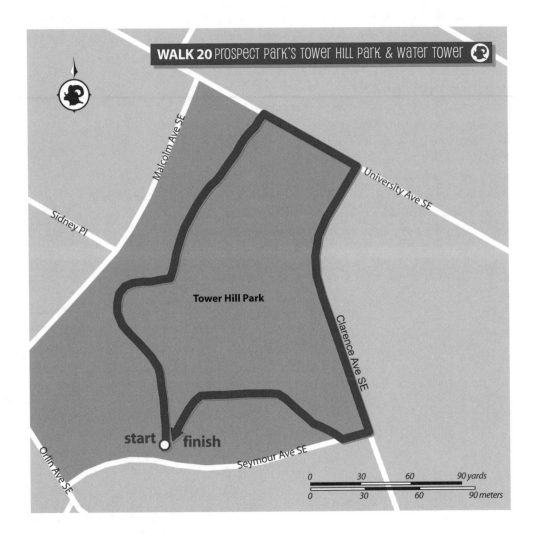

WALK 20 prospect park's tower hill park & water tower

Malcolm Ave SE

Sidney Pl

University Ave SE

Tower Hill Park

Clarence Ave SE

start ○ finish

Orlin Ave SE

Seymour Ave SE

| 0 | 30 | 60 | 90 yards |
| 0 | 30 | 60 | 90 meters |

20 Prospect Park's Tower Hill Park & Water Tower: Small Park, Scenic View

BOUNDARIES: Seymour Ave. S.E., Orlin Ave. S.E., Malcolm Ave. S.E., University Ave. S.E., Clarence Ave. S.E.

HUDSON'S TWIN CITY STREET ATLAS **COORDINATES: Map 394, 5C**

DISTANCE: Approx. ¾ mile

DIFFICULTY: Strenuous

PARKING: Free parking on the south side of Seymour Ave. S.E.

PUBLIC TRANSIT: Bus line 16

Prospect Park is an unusual neighborhood in Minneapolis, distinct in its piquant combination of hilly terrain, thick woods, and streets that weave throughout the upscale area. The hill that is today Tower Hill Park was created by a glacier 14,000 years ago. It was first settled in the 1880s, and the landmark Water Tower was erected in 1914. The housing stock has remained well preserved over the years, and the area is perennially home to academics from the nearby University of Minnesota.

The focal point of the neighborhood is Tower Hill Park and the scenic overlook that sits atop the summit. The brief, but strenuous, walk provides arguably the best scenic overlook of downtown Minneapolis. Pack a picnic lunch. Then after the challenging walk, enjoy dining alfresco where the views of nature and the city are synchronized seamlessly.

Warning: Walkers should exercise extreme caution when descending the steep hill, and avoid it entirely when snow and ice are on the ground, making the path slick and impassable.

- Begin by crossing Seymour Ave. S.E. and following the path that ascends the paved steps (closest to the tennis court) to the Water Tower.

- Take a left at the top of the stairs, just past the park bench.

- Continue straight ahead up the next set of stairs. On the right is the Water Tower (1914) and a plaque commemorating Minneapolis city engineer Frederick Cappelan's alluring and functional design. To the left of the tower, park benches allow you to take in incredible views of Minneapolis. In the immediate foreground is the rooftop of Pratt Community School. A small part of the current structure was built in 1898. It is the oldest Minneapolis public school building still serving its original purpose. Beyond the neighborhood is the University of Minnesota, and in the background is the downtown Minneapolis skyline—you'll notice the IDS Center, Wells Fargo Center, and Foshay Tower.

● Upon reaching the first exit in the observation area, take a left and follow the steep path that descends the hill. *Warning:* Do not attempt to follow this path in icy months. Instead, when the weather is uncooperative, follow the second left for a gentler descent down the hill.

● Continue following the edge of the woods downhill until you reach the sidewalk that runs parallel with University Ave. S.E.

● Turn right and follow the sidewalk that runs parallel with University Ave. Across the street are the radio and television towers for KSTP.

● Turn right and follow Clarence Ave. S.E. as it borders the park. The path steeply ascends the hill.

THE TOWER HILL OBSERVATION DECK: OPEN ONCE A YEAR

As if the panoramic view from Tower Hill wasn't exhilarating enough, the tower itself is open to the public during the annual Pratt Ice Cream Social. The event occurs the last week in May or the first week in June, thanks to the local neighborhood group Prospect Park East River Road Improvement Association. The ice cream social embraces the area's diversity, serving not only ice cream but also bratwurst, egg rolls, and *sambusas* (a Somali version of samosas) on the Pratt Community School grounds.

The observation deck of Tower Hill provides the highlight of the evening. Open for only 3 hours a year, it offers a breathtaking view of Minneapolis from the 107-foot-high concrete structure that locals refer to as the "witch's hat" because of its immense conical roof. The tower is a local landmark, and the event is not to be missed.

- Turn right on Seymour Ave. S.E. Across the street are examples of the neighborhood's diverse yet fully integrated architecture. The Lowell Lamoreaux House (39 Seymour Ave. S.E.) is a lovely example of Shingle style, with an unusual granite porch. On this block modern and large Victorian homes fit together surprisingly well.

- At the corner, turn right immediately onto the park path and follow it up the hill for another gorgeous view of the Water Tower.

- Turn left at the fork in front of the Water Tower.

- Turn left on the stairs and descend the path to return to Seymour Ave. S.E., our starting point.

POINT OF INTEREST

Tower Hill Park and Water Tower pperr.org/history/thetower.html, 55 Malcolm Ave. S.E., Minneapolis, MN 55414

ROUTE SUMMARY

1. Begin by crossing Seymour Ave. S.E. and following the path that ascends the paved steps to the Water Tower.
2. At the top of the stairs, take a left at the park bench.
3. Continue straight ahead up the next set of stairs.
4. Take a left upon reaching the first exit from the observation area. Follow the steep path that descends the hill.
5. Continue following the edge of the woods downhill until it reaches the sidewalk that runs parallel with University Ave. S.E.
6. Turn right at the sidewalk that runs parallel with University Ave.
7. Turn right and follow Clarence Ave. S.E. as it borders the park.
8. Turn right on Seymour Ave. S.E.
9. At the corner, take an immediate right on the park path and follow it up the hill.
10. Turn left at the fork in front of the Water Tower.
11. Turn left on the stairs and descend the path to return to Seymour Ave. S.E. to finish the walk.

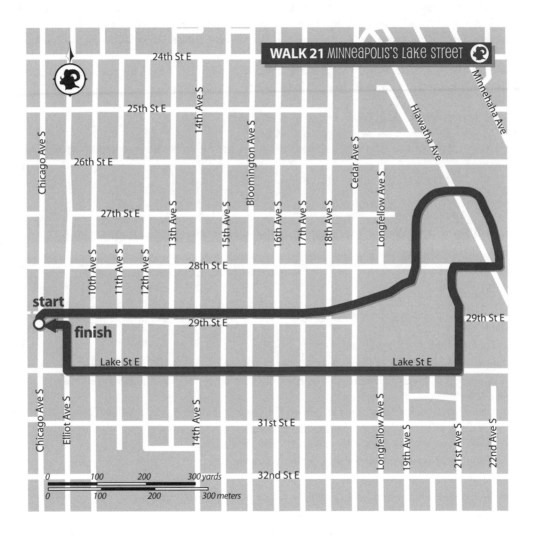

24th St E

25th St E

26th St E

27th St E

28th St E

29th St E

Lake St E

31st St E

32nd St E

29th St E

Lake St E

Chicago Ave S

Elliot Ave S

10th Ave S

11th Ave S

12th Ave S

13th Ave S

14th Ave S

15th Ave S

Bloomington Ave S

16th Ave S

17th Ave S

18th Ave S

Cedar Ave S

Longfellow Ave S

Hiawatha Ave

Minnehaha Ave

Longfellow Ave S

19th Ave S

21st Ave S

22nd Ave S

14th Ave S

start

finish

0   100   200   300 yards

0   100   200   300 meters

21 MINNEAPOLIS'S LAKE STREET: RICH IN CULTURES & HISTORY

BOUNDARIES: Lake St. E., Chicago Ave. S., 26th St. E., Minnehaha Ave.
HUDSON'S TWIN CITY STREET ATLAS **COORDINATES: Map 394, 3D and 4D**
DISTANCE: Approx. 3 miles
DIFFICULTY: Moderate
PARKING: Free 3-hour parking at the 10th Ave. S. Parking Ramp with validation at the Midtown Global Market
PUBLIC TRANSIT: Numerous bus lines to Transit Center

This walk will take you through one of the most culturally vibrant and constantly changing sections of Minneapolis. The two crown jewels of the neighborhood are longtime-resident Mercado Central and the much newer Midtown Global Market. Mercado Central was one of the first Latino marketplaces in the area, and many local Latino restaurateurs got their start renting a space in the mini-mall. Midtown Global Market is a cultural center representing more than two dozen countries and ethnic groups, with restaurants serving authentic dishes from Mexico, Vietnam, Japan, Sweden, the Middle East, and Somalia, to name a few, as well as pan-fusion gourmet food that transcends borders. Vending kiosks offer clothes, jewelry, toys, knickknacks, and specialty deli and dessert items from just as many countries.

● Start at the Transit Center just off the corner of Lake St. E. and Chicago Ave. S. Across the street from here is Uncle Hugo's Science Fiction Bookstore (the oldest independent science-fiction bookstore in the country) and Uncle Edgar's Mystery Bookstore.

● Go straight past the Transit Center, heading away from Lake St. E., and turn right at the first short set of stairs. Go down to the bottom of the big staircase and turn right onto the Midtown Greenway. To your left is Freewheel Bike, where you can either buy a new bike or fix up your old one.

● Go straight along the greenway approximately 1¼ miles until you get to 28th St. E. You'll see that navigating through Minneapolis via the greenway is easy, as street signs are located all along the path, and access to the upper street level can be found every quarter mile.

● Cross 28th St. E. at the crosswalk and take the left path.

● Continue over the Martin Olav Sabo Bridge, named after the Minnesota Congressman. The design for this amazing cable-style bridge came from drawings first rendered by Croatian inventor Faust Vrancic in his book *Machinae Novae*, published in 1595. This is the first bridge in the country to be successfully built to Vrancic's design specifications. The Hiawatha light-rail line runs directly underneath the bridge.

● Take the first right to cross Hiawatha Ave. and go straight west to follow 28th St. E. To your left is Eco-Yard Midtown, a prairie grassland restoration area and butterfly garden.

● Turn left at 21st Ave. S. and go south. This path takes you past the Green Institute, a non-profit design group that creates green-friendly building materials. Another prairie restoration project is along this path—this one filled with native grasses and wildflowers.

● Cross 29th St. E. and continue south.

● Turn right at Lake St. E. This path parallels the Minneapolis Pioneers and Soldiers Memorial Cemetery, the oldest cemetery in Minneapolis. The land originally belonged to a man named Martin Layman (hence the original name, Layman's Cemetery), who began using the grounds for pauper burials in the 1850s. The cemetery was eventually closed in 1919 due to neglect, and remained so until Minneapolis bought the grounds in 1928. Approximately 20,000 people are buried here, with only a quarter of the graves marked. A glimpse through the iron grates reveals ancient oak trees and weathered stone gravestones—some toppled over or broken beyond repair—marked by barely legible dates. The historic cemetery is open April 15–October 15.

● Cross 16th Ave. S. and keep going straight. Across the street and to your left is Ingebretsen's Scandinavian Gifts, which was founded in 1921 and remains the last operating vestige of that era. Formerly in disrepair, the neighborhood has seen new life, thanks to investments made by Latino business owners since the 1990s. Guayaquil serves Ecuadorian food, including many tempting seafood dishes. Inside

THE MIDTOWN GREENWAY: CONNECTING THE MISSISSIPPI RIVER TO UPTOWN

Opened in 2007, the Midtown Greenway is a combination bicycle and pedestrian path built on the remnants of the abandoned Milwaukee Road railway lines that once ran through the trench you're in now. The greenway is currently a little more than 5 miles long, but many, many more miles will be open to the public in the years ahead. Because of its location, pedestrians and cyclists can make their way through one of the busiest sections of south Minneapolis without having to stop for—or, for the most part, even *see*—a single car. Instead, travelers on the greenway are treated to community gardens, public art, and an underside view of dozens of historic bridges. The greenway is open 24 hours a day to commuters and is well lit at night, with emergency police call boxes located at regular intervals along the path. During the winter, the path is regularly plowed to make it easily accessible for the die-hard pedestrians and bicyclists who brave the route even in the coldest months.

Mercado Central is Taqueria La Hacienda, home of the best tacos in town.

● On the corner of 15th Ave. S. and Lake St. E. is In the Heart of the Beast Puppet and Mask Theatre. Every spring, the theater puts on a May Day parade that features bigger-than-life papier-mâché puppets portraying everything from butterflies and pagan goddesses to the latest figures in politics. The theater is also famous for contributing puppets to celebrations and political protest marches around the world.

● Continue west down Lake St. and turn right on Elliot Ave. S. To your right is the Midtown Global Market, the jewel of this neighborhood. Located inside the former Sears building, dozens of kiosks sell deli items and merchandise from local farmers and international merchants, while some of the best restaurants in the Twin Cities have set up miniature offshoots here. Some of the can't-miss places include Tibet Arts & Gifts, with handmade textiles and jewelry at reasonable prices; Café Finspäng, which carries Scandinavian foods, books, and gifts; Panaderia El Mexicano, home of some of the prettiest cakes and tastiest flan in town; Manny's Tortas, which sells just-as-spicy-as-you-like-'em sandwiches; Salty Tart, which carries cakes and cookies way too good to share; La Loma, considered to be the home of the best tamales in town by just about every restaurant critic in the Twin Cities;

and Los Ocampo, which makes Mexican food so authentic that many of the recipes are derived from 6,000-year-old Aztec delights.

● Turn left by the parking lot to reach the Transit Center, the starting point.

POINTS OF INTEREST

Uncle Hugo's/Uncle Edgar's unclehugo.com, 2864 Chicago Ave. S., Minneapolis, MN 55407, 612-824-6347/612-824-9984

Midtown Greenway midtowngreenway.org, Abbott Ave. S. to W. River Pkwy. along Lake St. E., Minneapolis, MN 55416 and 55406, 612-879-0103

Freewheel Bike freewheelbike.com, 2834 10th Ave. S., Minneapolis, MN 55407, 612-238-4447

Eco-Yard Midtown hennepin.us/ecoyardtours, 22801 21st Ave. S., Minneapolis, MN 55407, 612-348-3777

Minneapolis Pioneers and Soldiers Memorial Cemetery friendsofthecemetery.org, 2945 Cedar Ave. S., Minneapolis, MN 55407, 612-729-8484

Ingebretsen's Scandinavian Gifts ingebretsens.com, 1601 Lake St. E., Minneapolis, MN 55407, 612-729-9333

Guayaquil 1526 Lake St. E., Minneapolis, MN 55407, 612-722-2346

Mercado Central mercadocentral.net, 1515 Lake St. E., Minneapolis, MN 55407, 612-728-5401

Taqueria La Hacienda taquerialahacienda.com, 1515 Lake St. E., #104, Minneapolis, MN 55407, 612-822-2715

In the Heart of the Beast Puppet and Mask Theatre hobt.org, 1500 Lake St. E., Minneapolis, MN 55407, 612-721-2535

Midtown Global Market midtownglobalmarket.org, 2929 Chicago Ave. S., Minneapolis, MN 55407, 612-872-4041

route summary

1. Start at the Transit Center near the corner of Lake St. E. and Chicago Ave. S.
2. Turn right at the first short set of stairs past the Transit Center and go down to the bottom of the big staircase.
3. Turn right onto the Midtown Greenway and follow it until you cross 28th St. E.
4. Take the left path to cross Martin Olav Sabo Bridge.
5. Take your first right to cross Hiawatha Ave. and go straight to follow 28th St. E.
6. Turn left at the corner of 21st Ave. S. and go straight south.
7. Turn right on Lake St. E.
8. Turn right on Elliot Ave. S.
9. Turn left by the parking lot to reach the Transit Center, our starting point.

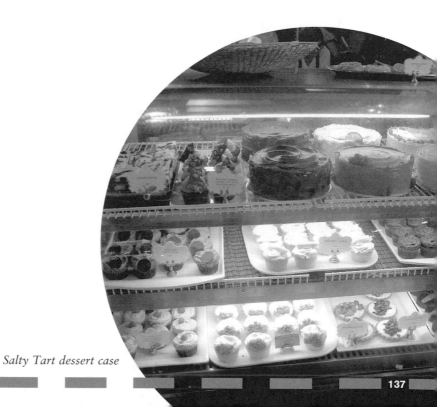

Salty Tart dessert case

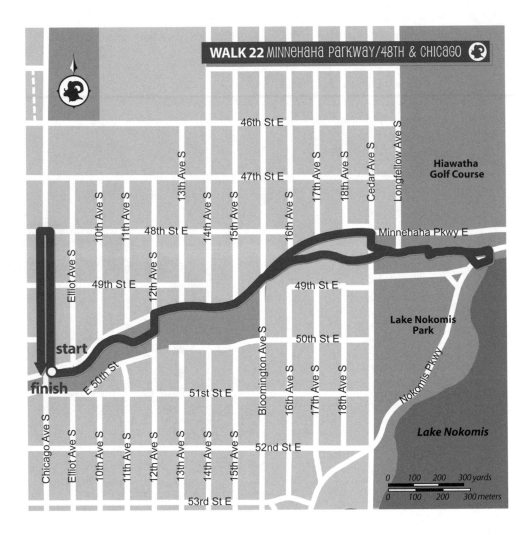

WALK 22 MINNEHAHA PARKWAY/48TH & CHICAGO

46th St E

47th St E

13th Ave S

Hiawatha
Golf Course

17th Ave S
18th Ave S
Cedar Ave S
Longfellow Ave S

10th Ave S
11th Ave S
48th St E
14th Ave S
15th Ave S
16th Ave S

Minnehaha Pkwy E

Elliot Ave S
12th Ave S

49th St E

49th St E

Lake Nokomis
Park

start

50th St E

Bloomington Ave S
16th Ave S
17th Ave S
18th Ave S

E 50th St

finish

Nokomis Pkwy

51st St E

Chicago Ave S
Elliot Ave S
10th Ave S
11th Ave S
12th Ave S
13th Ave S
14th Ave S
15th Ave S

52nd St E

Lake Nokomis

0   100   200   300 yards
0   100   200   300 meters

53rd St E

22 MINNEHAHA PARKWAY/48TH & CHICAGO: Green space, relaxation space

BOUNDARIES: **Minnehaha Pkwy. E., Chicago Ave. S., 48th St. E., Nokomis Pkwy.**
HUDSON'S TWIN CITY STREET ATLAS **COORDINATES: Map 421, 3B and 4B**
DISTANCE: Approx. 3 miles
DIFFICULTY: Moderate
PARKING: Free parking on Chicago Ave. S. and Minnehaha Pkwy. E.
PUBLIC TRANSIT: Bus line 22

Three of the city's landmarks rich in natural geography combine for this walk: first, a lovely section of the Grand Rounds, Minnehaha Pkwy.; second, a charming business district, 48th St. and Chicago in McRae Park; and finally, a lake, Lake Nokomis. The proximity of nature and small town–like business districts is relatively common in the Twin Cities, but this walk stands out. Minnehaha Pkwy. is one of the seven byway districts in Minneapolis's Grand Rounds Scenic Byway. Minnehaha Park passes through the neighborhood en route to Minnehaha Falls a few miles away, and just over the hill lies a quaint and quirky shopping district with numerous independently owned businesses. Nothing could be better on a hot summer day than enjoying a delicious organic ice cream at the Pumphouse Creamery after exploring the parkway and Lake Nokomis.

The scenic pathways on Minnehaha Pkwy. are slightly confusing, so pay close attention to the directions and map. Also, paths are divided into bicycle-only, pedestrian-only, and combined categories. Parts of this walk are on the combined path—be aware of bicyclists zooming by, but most important, relax and enjoy the fresh air.

● **Begin at the southeast corner of Chicago Ave. S. and Minnehaha Pkwy. E. and walk south, crossing Minnehaha Creek.**

● **Turn left immediately on the first path that wends through the woods, walking toward the east. Jets can be heard overhead on their way to and from nearby Minneapolis–St. Paul International Airport.**

- Turn left on the path that follows Minnehaha Creek, and take another left at 12th Ave. S. to cross the stone bridge.

- Cross 12th Ave. S., and then turn right on Minnehaha Pkwy. E. Follow the pedestrian path east along the creek, where a wetland restoration project is in place to prevent further erosion and improve water quality.

- Continue to the east along the creek after the path intersects. Take in the wild irises and native plants ahead. The pedestrian and bike paths merge before Bloomington Ave. S., so be careful here.

- Go straight, continuing east, after crossing Bloomington Ave. S., and then go right as the path follows the creek. Continue following the winding path lined with pines, willows, and oaks.

- Continue straight at the intersection with the bridge, and at the fork ahead, stay next to the creek. This part of the parkway is swampy lowland with reeds, red-winged blackbirds, and an abundance of flora and fauna.

- After passing under the Cedar Avenue Bridge, continue along the creek.

- Continue straight until reaching the parking lot and information kiosk at 2125 Minnehaha Ave.; then turn right to cross the pedestrian bridge.

- Continue forward, carefully crossing Nokomis Pkwy., and turn left to follow the pedestrian path as it curves along the lake. Lake Nokomis Beach can be seen to the south through the trees.

- Cross the bridge; then after approximately 100 feet turn left on the pedestrian path and carefully cut across the bike path and Nokomis Pkwy. In the opposite direction, about a quarter mile ahead on Nokomis Pkwy., are the Nokomis Community Center and public restrooms.

- After crossing Nokomis Pkwy., follow the pedestrian path, and then turn left to cross the concrete bridge. On the left is the lock that the city can adjust to control the water level of Lake Nokomis—either stopping the water to fill the lake, or allowing it to flow down the creek.

● Turn left on the pedestrian path after passing the kiosk and parking lot again.

● Turn right on the pedestrian path before going under the Cedar Avenue S. Bridge. Follow the path to the corner of Cedar Ave. S. and cross Minnehaha Pkwy. E.

● Continue across Cedar Ave. S. and turn right across Minnehaha Pkwy. E. Walk to the sidewalk of the service road and turn left, headed west. The neighborhood is a lovely, tree-shaded residential area.

● Continue west on Minnehaha Pkwy. E. after crossing Bloomington Ave. S., where an eclectic architecture collection—from Tudors to modern eco-homes—lines the parkway.

● Turn right on Chicago Ave. S. and proceed up the steep hill toward the McRae Park business district.

● Continue on Chicago Ave. S., descending the hill. Take in the view that overlooks the business district and drop in for something sweet at Candy Alley.

● After crossing 48th St. E. turn left, and turn left again to walk in the opposite direction on Chicago Ave. S. Shop in the City is a locally run store with a great selection of gifts, home décor, jewelry, and local souvenirs. North of 48th St. E. on Chicago Ave. S. is arguably the Twin

Candy Alley

Cities best ice cream parlor, Pumphouse Creamery, where a rotating selection of 20 organic ice creams and sorbets delights the taste buds—whether strawberry, banana, or mouthwatering local cherry. A few doors down is one of three locations of the local leader in baking, the Turtle Bread Company. Since 1994, it has offered up fresh breads, cakes, pies, cookies, and pastries, as well as sandwiches, homemade soups, and breakfast. Just around the corner is Café Levain, a reasonably priced neighborhood bistro with a rotating menu that might include mussels and beef spareribs.

● After crossing 48th St. E. you'll come to another block of fine foods and entertainment. First is Town Hall Tap, with excellent beer crafted in-house and equally excellent food. On the right is Pepito's Parkway Theater: a collaboration between two local mainstays, Pepito's Mexican Restaurant and the Pepito's Parkway Theater (1931). Since its inception in 1971, Pepito's has served Mexican American favorites such as tacos, enchiladas, burritos, and even chicken mole in an incredibly friendly and cozy environment. The Parkway was recently purchased by Pepito's and now serves beer, wine, and food.

● Continue to ascend and then descend Chicago Ave. S. to finish the walk.

POINTS OF INTEREST

Lake Nokomis tinyurl.com/lakenokomis, 4955 W. Lake Nokomis Pkwy., Minneapolis, MN 55417, 612-370-4923

Candy Alley candyalley.com, 4817 Chicago Ave. S., Minneapolis, MN 55417, 612-354-3881

Shop in the City 4737 Chicago Ave. S., Minneapolis, MN 55407, 612-825-2808

Pumphouse Creamery pumphouse-creamery.com, 4754 Chicago Ave. S., Minneapolis, MN 55407, 612-825-2021

Turtle Bread Company turtlebread.com, 4782 Chicago Ave. S., Minneapolis, MN 55407, 612-823-7333

Café Levain cafelevain.com, 4762 Chicago Ave. S., Minneapolis, MN 55407, 612-823-7111

Horace W. S. Cleveland:
Father of the Grand Rounds National Scenic Byway

In the fledgling days of Minneapolis, landscape architect Horace W. S. Cleveland (1814–1900) had a keen sense of foresight, predicting the rise of a great city and recognizing the importance of purchasing parklands for public use. Cleveland finished second to Frederick Law Olmsted in his design for Central Park in New York City but found success with his public designs elsewhere. His later civil engineering accomplishments include the parkway system in Omaha, Nebraska, and Sleepy Hollow Cemetery in Concord, Massachusetts.

The Grand Rounds, a linked series of park areas, are some of Minneapolis's greatest civic assets. The byway runs through seven districts: the Mississippi River, Theodore Wirth, Northeast, Chain of Lakes, Victory Memorial, Downtown Riverfront, and Minnehaha. With 50.1 miles, and more land being acquired for walking, biking, and driving, this system is recognized as one of the nation's best. The Minnehaha byway is 12.8 miles of multiuse green space and parkway along the creek. Cleveland's legacy is felt daily by Minneapolitans enjoying the city's extensive scenic byways.

Town Hall Tap townhallbrewery.com, 4810 Chicago Ave. S., Minneapolis, MN 55407, 612-767-7307

Pepito's Mexican Restaurant pepitosrestaurant.com, 4820 Chicago Ave. S., Minneapolis, MN 55417, 612-822-2104

Pepito's Parkway Theater theparkwaytheater.com, 4814 Chicago Ave. S., Minneapolis, MN 55417, 612-822-3030

route summary

1. Begin at the southeast corner of Chicago Ave. S. and Minnehaha Pkwy. E. and walk south, crossing Minnehaha Creek.

2. Turn left immediately on the first path that wends through the woods, walking east.

3. Turn left on the path that follows Minnehaha Creek. At 12th Ave. S., turn left to cross the stone bridge.

4. Turn right on Minnehaha Pkwy. E. after crossing 12th Ave. S., following the pedestrian path along the creek.

5. Continue to the east along the creek after the path intersects.

6. Continue after crossing Bloomington Ave. S., and then turn right as the path follows along the creek.

7. Continue straight at the intersection with the bridge. At the fork ahead, stay next to the creek.

8. After passing under the Cedar Avenue Bridge, continue along the creek.

9. Continue straight until reaching the parking lot and information kiosk at 2125 Minnehaha Ave.; then turn right to cross the pedestrian bridge.

10. Carefully cross Nokomis Pkwy., and turn left to follow the pedestrian path as it curves along the lake.

11. Cross the bridge, and then after approximately 100 feet turn left on the pedestrian path and carefully cut across the bike path and Nokomis Pkwy.

12. Follow the pedestrian path, turn left, and cross the concrete bridge.

13. Turn left on the pedestrian path after passing the kiosk and parking lot again.

14. Turn right on the pedestrian path before going under the Cedar Avenue Bridge. Follow the path to the corner of Cedar Ave. S. and cross Minnehaha Pkwy. E.

15. Cross Cedar Ave. S. and turn right across Minnehaha Pkwy. E. Walk to the sidewalk of the service road and turn left, heading west.

16. Continue west on Minnehaha Pkwy. E. after crossing Bloomington Ave. S.

17. Turn right on Chicago Ave. S.

18. After crossing 48th St. E. turn left, and turn left again to walk in the opposite direction on Chicago Ave. S.

19. Continue to ascend and then descend Chicago Ave. S. to finish the walk.

Minnehaha Parkway

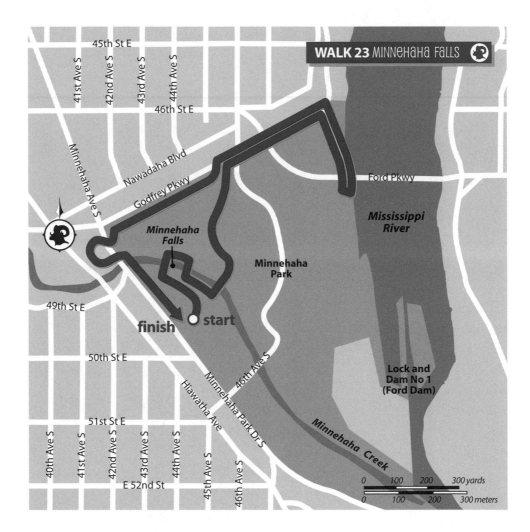

45th St E

41st Ave S

42nd Ave S

43rd Ave S

44th Ave S

46th St E

Minnehaha Ave S

Nawadaha Blvd

Godfrey Pkwy

Ford Pkwy

Mississippi River

Minnehaha Falls

Minnehaha Park

49th St E

finish ● **start**

50th St E

Minnehaha Park Dr S

46th Ave S

Hiawatha Ave

Lock and Dam No 1 (Ford Dam)

51st St E

40th Ave S

41st Ave S

42nd Ave S

43rd Ave S

44th Ave S

45th Ave S

46th Ave S

E 52nd St

Minnehaha Creek

0   100   200   300 yards

0   100   200   300 meters

23 MINNEHAHA FALLS: "OF THE LOVELY LAUGHING WATERS"

BOUNDARIES: **50th St. E., Hiawatha Ave., Godfrey Pkwy., Mississippi River**
HUDSON'S TWIN CITY STREET ATLAS COORDINATES: **Map 421, 5B; Map 422, 1B**
DISTANCE: **Approx. 2¼ miles**
DIFFICULTY: **Moderate**
PARKING: **Free parking on Minnehaha Ave. S.**
PUBLIC TRANSIT: **Light-rail at the 50th St. Minnehaha Park Station**

If you're a fan of Henry Wadsworth Longfellow's poetry, or simply interested in 19th-century Americana in general, then a stop at Minnehaha Falls is an absolute must. The falls, which share the name of Longfellow's tragically fated heroine and translate from the Dakota to mean "laughing waters," were a major tourist attraction long before the area was designated as parkland in 1883. In the spring and summer, visitors are treated to picturesque waterfalls cascading over a tree-lined chasm and into Minnehaha Creek below; in the wintertime, the falls are frozen into glistening blue, white, and green gigantic icicles. They're probably not the tallest waterfalls you'll ever see, but they are unique in their surroundings—an exquisite park with waterfalls, wildflowers, sandstone cliffs, and big, open wilderness spaces, all located in the heart of a busy metropolis.

Note: During the winter, all the staircases leading to the bottom of the falls are closed. It's still worth a visit to see the frozen waterfalls from the top, even if you can't get down to the lower paths.

● Start in front of the John Harrington Stevens House. It's the little white house in the park, located right off of Minnehaha Park Dr. and 50th St. E. Built in 1850, it was Minneapolis's very first house. It was originally where the downtown Minneapolis Post Office building is now but was moved here in 1890; after eventually being refurbished, it reopened to the public in the 1980s.

● Facing the Stevens House, turn left to head into the park. This route takes you under the canopy of the vine-covered pergola. Native plants and flowers, including trilliums, wood poppies, and columbines surround both sides of the structure. The right side looks out over the bluffs leading down to Minnehaha Creek.

- Go straight past the first set of stairs and go down the second set to your right. You are now walking directly over the top of Minnehaha Falls. If you look to the left while crossing the bridge, you'll get a glimpse of the bronze statue commemorating the love of Hiawatha and Minnehaha.

- Turn right at the bottom of the stairs. Follow the retaining wall until you get to the next set of stairs, located on your right. Before heading down the stairs, stop and take a look at the falls. From way up here, you get a spectacular view of them cascading into Minnehaha Creek below, as well as the grotto hollowed out by the pounding force of the water. Behind you is the picnic pavilion, which has indoor tables, restrooms, water fountains, soda machines, and bicycle rentals. The pavilion is also home to Sea Salt Eatery, one of the best seafood restaurants in the Twin Cities.

- Go all the way down to the bottom of the winding staircase and turn right. This spot offers the best view of the scope of Minnehaha Falls. The stairs and masonry along this path were initiated by the Works Progress Administration in the 1930s.

- Turn left to cross the little stone bridge, and make another left onto the dirt path. This path follows the course of Minnehaha Creek, to your left; notice the amazing limestone and sandstone cliffs on the right.

- At the next bridge, take the far-right path into the woods. This area is home to some of Minnesota's most beautiful wildflowers, including orchidlike, orange-spotted touch-me-nots and tiny blue-and-yellow forget-me-nots.

- Turn left at the bridge. Off to the right of the bridge you'll see a boardwalk path leading into the woods. If you're feeling adventurous, take this one-way path to the banks of the Mississippi River. However, it's very rustic and often flooded in the springtime and any time after a heavy rainstorm.

- Cross the bridge and take a left at the fork.

- At the next fork, take the left path to follow the creek.

● Turn left to go down the hill. Here's where the path ends. If the weather's warm and you feel like taking a dip, the water is refreshing and rarely more than knee-deep, making it a popular wading spot for park-goers.

● Turn right to go through the grassy field. At the far end of the field, you'll see a graded path that you'll want to take uphill.

● At the top of the hill, turn right.

● At the next fork, turn left.

● At the corner next to the VETERANS HOME sign at 46th Ave. S., turn right to cross the street.

● Go straight to follow Godfrey Pkwy. on the combined bicycle/pedestrian path. On your left and right are prairie restoration areas, where wildflowers such as daylilies, coneflowers, daisies, and prairie grass have been planted.

● Go under the bridge and keep going straight.

● Take the first right and cross the parking lot to the UPPER MISSISSIPPI RIVER LOCKS AND DAMS NO. 1 sign.

● Turn right to go down the hill and under the Ford Bridge. This path takes you close to the Mississippi River and its neighboring bluffs.

● Go down to Ford Dam/Locks and Dam No. 1 Promenade. From here, you can see the locks and dam to your

Minnehaha Falls

right, while across the river are the buff-colored buildings of the Ford Hydroelectric Plant. You can fish off the steps here if you have a fishing license.

● Turn around and follow the path to the right, back to the top of the hill. Go straight until you reach the Park & Recreation Board kiosk. This sign has information about the history and purpose of the locks and dams you just saw.

● Turn left and go straight to cross the Locks & Dams No. 1 entrance road. Continue straight to go under the bridge.

● At the end of the block, take the left fork. Go straight to continue following Godfrey Pkwy.

● Keep following the path around, past the playground and to the front parking lot. When the path splits, turn left.

● Follow the path and cross Minnehaha Ave.

● Turn right. The yellow house to your left is the Longfellow House, a two-thirds-scale replica of Henry Wadsworth Longfellow's house in Cambridge, Massachusetts. Robert "Fish" Jones, famous fishmonger, showman, and entrepreneur, was a huge Longfellow fan and had the house built in 1906. Over the years, the house has served as a zoo, library, haunted house, and, in its current role, as an office for the Park Board.

● Follow the path around the house and up the hill.

● Turn left into Longfellow Gardens. Take the next immediate left and follow the path through the garden. Longfellow Gardens was also run by Fish Jones, who used the grounds as a zoo, amusement park, and formal gardens.

● When you're done in the gardens, head toward the staircase by the Longfellow House. Go down the stairs and straight to cross the train tracks.

● Go straight and cross Minnehaha Ave. S., and then turn right to follow Minnehaha Park Dr. S.

- Across the street is the Minnehaha Depot, a little brown train depot that is also called the Princess Depot because of its dainty size and design. Built in 1875, the depot was one of three stops on Minnesota's first railroad and, in its heyday, handled nearly 40 trains a day. Today, it serves as a mini-museum for the park and the railway system.

- Directly ahead is the white Stevens House, the starting point.

POINTS OF INTEREST

John Harrington Stevens House johnhstevenshouse.org, 4901 Minnehaha Ave. S., Minneapolis, MN 55417, 612-722-2220

Minnehaha Park tinyurl.com/minnehahapark, 4801 Minnehaha Park Dr. S., Minneapolis, MN 55417, 612-230-6400

Sea Salt Eatery seasalteatery.wordpress.com, 4825 Minnehaha Ave. S., Minneapolis, MN 55417, 612-721-8990

Ford Dam/Upper Mississippi River Locks and Dams No. 1 mvp.usace.army.mil, 5000 Godfrey Pkwy., Minneapolis, MN 55417

Longfellow House tinyurl.com/houselongfellow, 4800 Minnehaha Ave. S., Minneapolis, MN 55417, 612-230-6520

Longfellow Gardens tinyurl.com/longfellowgardens, 3933 Minnehaha Pkwy. E., Minneapolis, MN 55417, 612-230-6400

Minnehaha/Princess Depot mtmuseum.org/mhdepot.shtml, 4801 Minnehaha Ave. S., Minneapolis, MN 55417, 612-230-6400

ROUTE SUMMARY

1. Start at the statue in front of the John Harrington Stevens House.
2. Turn left to head into the park. Go through the pergola.
3. Go straight and down the second set of stairs to your right.
4. Turn right at the bottom of the stairs. Follow the retaining wall until you get to the next set of stairs.
5. Go all the way down to the bottom of the winding staircase and turn right.

6. Turn left to cross the little stone bridge.

7. Make another left to follow the dirt path.

8. At the next bridge, take the far-right path into the woods.

9. Turn left at the bridge.

10. Cross the bridge and take a left at the fork.

11. At the next fork, take the left path.

12. Take the next left to go down the hill.

13. Turn right to go through the grassy field. Head for the path to your far right and go up the hill.

14. At the top of the hill, turn right.

15. At the next fork, turn left.

16. At the VETERANS HOME sign, turn right to cross the street.

17. Go straight to follow Godfrey Pkwy.

18. Take the first right and cross the parking lot to the UPPER MISSISSIPPI RIVER LOCKS AND DAMS NO. 1 sign.

19. Turn right to go down the hill and under the bridge.

20. Turn around and follow the path to the right, back to the top of the hill. Go straight until you reach the Park & Recreation Board kiosk.

21. Turn left and go straight. Cross the Locks & Dam No. 1 entrance road, and keep going straight.

22. At the end of the block, take the left fork. Go straight to continue following Godfrey Pkwy.

23. Keep following the path around to the front parking lot. When the path splits, turn left.

24. Go straight and cross Minnehaha Ave. S.

25. Turn right.

26. Follow the path around the house and up the hill, and turn left into Longfellow Gardens. Take the next immediate left and follow the path through the garden.

27. Head toward the staircase by the Longfellow House.

28. Go down the stairs and straight to cross the train tracks.

29. Go straight and cross Minnehaha Ave. S.

30. Turn right to follow Minnehaha Park Dr. S.

31. Go straight to return to the Stevens House and finish the walk.

Mask of Chief Little Crow

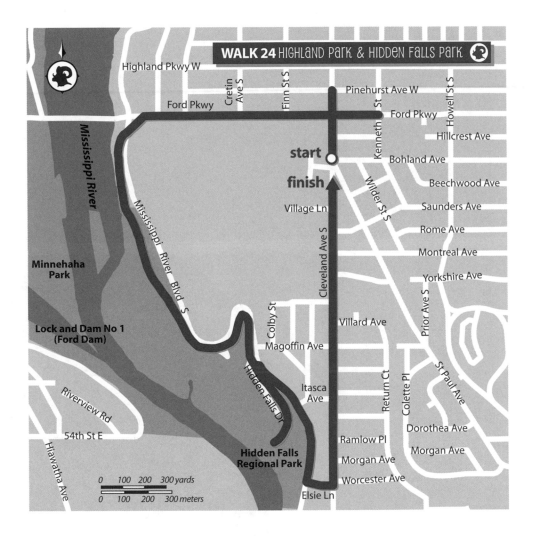

Highland Pkwy W

Ford Pkwy

Cretin Ave S

Finn St S

Pinehurst Ave W

Kenneth St

Ford Pkwy

Howell St S

Hillcrest Ave

start

Bohland Ave

Beechwood Ave

finish

Wilder St S

Saunders Ave

Village Ln

Rome Ave

Montreal Ave

Yorkshire Ave

Cleveland Ave S

Prior Ave S

Mississippi River

Mississippi River Blvd S

Minnehaha Park

Lock and Dam No 1
(Ford Dam)

Colby St

Villard Ave

Magoffin Ave

Return Ct

Colette Pl

St Paul Ave

Hidden Falls Dr

Itasca Ave

Riverview Rd

54th St E

Hidden Falls
Regional Park

Ramlow Pl

Dorothea Ave

Morgan Ave

Morgan Ave

Hiawatha Ave

Worcester Ave

Elsie Ln

0   100   200   300 yards

0   100   200   300 meters

24 HIGHLAND PARK & HIDDEN FALLS PARK: NATURE, SHOPPING, & DINING

BOUNDARIES: **Mississippi River, Pinehurst Ave. W., Kenneth St., Elsie Ln.**
HUDSON'S TWIN CITY STREET ATLAS **COORDINATES: Map 422, 1B, 2B, and 1C**
DISTANCE: Approx. 4½ miles
DIFFICULTY: Moderate
PARKING: Free parking on Cleveland Ave.
PUBLIC TRANSIT: Bus lines 87 and 134

Highland Park is one of St. Paul's most affluent neighborhoods. It has an abundance of natural and cultural amenities, thanks to its location atop an idyllic bluff east of the Mississippi River and its diverse population. The Ford Twin Cities Assembly Plant, which called the area home since 1925, closed in 2012. Minnesota baseball legends who played or lived in the area as kids include Jack Morris, Dave Winfield, Paul Molitor, and Joe Mauer, 2006 American League Batting Champion of the Minnesota Twins. Highland Park is also a historic neighborhood for St. Paul's Jewish population, including Orthodox and Lubavitch Hasidim groups.

Beneath the surface of this upscale community, however, lie an unusually large number of famous crimes—from its origins as a Prohibition-era drinking stop and gangster hangout to St. Paul's most infamous murder, the 1963 T. Eugene Thompson case. A more recent high-profile example is that of Sara Jane Olson, also known as Kathleen Soliah in the Symbionese Liberation Army, who pled guilty in 2001 to possessing explosives with intent to murder, after living as a fugitive here for 23 years. This odd David Lynch–like juxtaposition of good and evil in Highland Park adds another dimension to an otherwise placid community.

● Begin at the southeast corner of Bohland Ave. and walk north on Cleveland Ave. S. On the right after crossing Hillcrest Ave. is Chatterbox Pub, a local favorite for burgers, pizza, good beer, and games, located in an unassuming former Perkins Family Restaurant.

● Turn right on Ford Pkwy. The Highland Village Center features local and national chain stores, plus a few neighborhood businesses. Highland Café and Bakery specializes in breakfast foods, such as waffles and omelets, as well as soups and sandwiches for lunch and dinner.

- Turn left on Kenneth St., and then turn left on Ford Pkwy., and return on the opposite side of Kenneth St. On the right, the Highland business district resumes at Half Price Books—an excellent national used-bookstore with a wide selection of inexpensive books, records, CDs, and DVDs for any taste.

- Turn right on Cleveland Ave. S., where the classic marquee of the Highland 2 Theatres dominates the comfy small-town feel of the street. On the right is TeaSource, premium purveyors of imported teas.

- Turn left at Pinehurst Ave. W., and immediately turn left again on Cleveland Ave. S., to return on the opposite side of Pinehurst Ave. W. This block includes excellent choices for anything from a small nosh and coffee to an all-you-can-eat buffet. Cleveland Wok falls into the latter category, with an extensive and inexpensive high-quality Chinese and Vietnamese buffet. Highland Grill serves American comfort food for breakfast, lunch, and dinner.

- Turn right on Ford Pkwy. The grade descends steeply after crossing Cretin Ave. S. The area on the left is the former Ford Motor Company production plant. The Ford Twin Cities Assembly Plant was constructed in 1925 to produce Model Ts and was later remodeled to accommodate technology changes in the auto-assembly industry. A 135-acre parcel of land overlooking the Mississippi River, the site presents a redevelopment challenge for Ford, the city of St. Paul, and the Highland Park neighborhood.

- Nearing the Mississippi River on Ford Pkwy., turn right on the path descending the hill next to the Intercity (Ford) Bridge—one of four concrete arch bridges linking Minneapolis and St. Paul.

- After carefully crossing Mississippi River Blvd., turn left. The path provides a breathtaking view of the river. Behind the sumac and in the river is Lock and Dam No. 1, most commonly known as Ford Dam. Constructed in 1917, the concrete dam is 574 feet long and 30 feet high. The dam played an important role in the effort to improve the once nearly impassable Mississippi River between downtown St. Paul and Minneapolis. Next to the dam is the hydroelectric plant, which Ford recently sold to Brookfield Power, a Canadian energy firm. Originally built to supply power for the assembly plant, the hydroelectric plant was a significant factor in luring Ford to the neighborhood in the '20s.

- Follow the path on the right to the Ford Dam Scenic Overlook, where you have a phenomenal vista on the Mississippi River. Across the river are several of the 22 Minnesota Historic Veterans Home buildings. The first eight were constructed as early as 1888 in the Richardsonian Romanesque style. The 51-acre VA Home sits nestled on the Mississippi, surrounded by Minnehaha Park.

- Continue approximately half a mile, following the pedestrian path on the bluff above the river through a vast network of forests and floodplains.

- Turn right on the pedestrian path on Mississippi River Blvd., curving around the falls, which become increasingly louder as you approach them. Before reaching the falls on the right is an excellent—though barely visible from the path—scenic overlook down a flight of stone steps.

- Continue on the path, passing Hidden Falls and approaching the park.

- Turn right after crossing Hidden Falls Dr., and descend the steep pedestrian path on the street.

- Continue following the path downhill. The picnic pavilion and public restrooms are to the right across the street.

- Continue following the path south as it snakes below the bluff, and turn left as the path forks. On the right is the Mississippi River and public boat access.

- Turn around and return in the opposite direction after taking in the river view. The Crosby Farm/Hidden Falls Regional Park, which comprises more than 130 acres and 6.7 miles of trails, merits its own nature walk.

- Continue to follow the path north along the river bluff and turn right when the path forks, to ascend the steep grade.

- At the top of the hill, turn right on Mississippi River Blvd. Look down the hill at Hidden Falls Regional Park. The view along this path is truly breathtaking; take a moment to look across the river at Fort Snelling and watch the planes at Minneapolis–St. Paul International Airport.

- Turn left on Elsie Ln. as it crosses the working-class residential area, Highland Park. In the late 1830s, four homes in this then-secluded area across the river from Fort Snelling formed Old Rum Town, where soldiers, trappers, and other transients imbibed clandestine cocktails. However, the homes on this block were built in the mid-20th century and lack a sidewalk, so walk carefully on this quiet neighborhood street.

- Turn left on Cleveland Ave. S. This section of Highland Park contains well-maintained, modest homes.

- Continue north, crossing the railroad bridge. On the left is the Ford Little League Park, where Minnesota Twins catcher Joe Mauer, three-time 20-game winner Jack Morris, former Minnesota Vikings Pro-Bowl center Matt Birk, and countless other kids played baseball. The baseball park closed because of high arsenic levels in 2007 but reopened in spring 2008.

- Head north on Cleveland Ave. S. to finish the walk. On the right are the lovely Highland Village Apartments, 12 Colonial Revival–style apartments.

POINTS OF INTEREST

Chatterbox Pub chatterboxpub.net, 800 Cleveland Ave. S., St. Paul, MN 55116, 651-699-1149

Highland Village Center tinyurl.com/highlandctr, 2024 Ford Pkwy., St. Paul, MN 55116

Highland Café & Bakery highlandcafeonline.com, 2012 Ford Pkwy., St. Paul, MN 55116, 651-698-3400

Half Price Books hpb.com, 2041 Ford Pkwy., St. Paul, MN 55116, 651-699-1391

Highland 2 Theatres manntheatresmn.com, 760 Cleveland Ave. S., St. Paul, MN 55116, 651-698-3085

TeaSource teasource.com, 752 Cleveland Ave. S., St. Paul, MN 55116, 651-690-9822

Cleveland Wok clevelandwok.com, 767 Cleveland Ave. S., St. Paul, MN 55116, 651-699-3141

Highland Grill highlandgrill.com, 771 Cleveland Ave. S., St. Paul, MN 55116, 651-690-1173

Ford Dam/Upper Mississippi River Locks and Dams No. 1 mvp.usace.army.mil, 5000 Godfrey Pkwy., Minneapolis, MN 55417

Hidden Falls Park tinyurl.com/hiddenfallsmn, 1313 Hidden Falls Dr., St. Paul, MN 55116, 651-632-5111

route summary

1. Begin at the southeast corner of Bohland Ave. and continue north on Cleveland Ave. S.

2. Turn right on Ford Pkwy.

3. Turn left on Kenneth Ave., and then turn left on Ford Pkwy., and return on the opposite side of the street.

4. Turn right on Cleveland Ave. S.

5. Turn left at Pinehurst Ave. W., and immediately turn left again on Cleveland Ave. S. to return on the opposite side of the street.

6. Turn right on Ford Pkwy.

7. Nearing the Mississippi River on Ford Pkwy., turn right on the path descending the hill next to the Intercity (Ford) Bridge.

8. Cross Mississippi River Blvd. and turn left.

9. Follow the path on the right.

10. Follow the pedestrian path south for approximately half a mile.

11. Turn right on the pedestrian path.

12. Continue on the path, passing Hidden Falls and approaching the park.

13. Turn right after crossing Hidden Falls Dr., and descend the steep pedestrian path of the street.

14. Continue following the path downhill.

15. Continue following the path as it snakes below the bluff, and turn left as the path forks.

16. Turn around and return in the opposite direction.

17. Continue following the path north along the river bluff, and turn right when the path forks.

18. At the top of the hill, go right on Mississippi River Blvd.

19. Turn left on Elsie Ln.

20. Turn left on Cleveland Ave. S.

21. Continue north, crossing the railroad bridge.

22. Head north on Cleveland Ave. S. to finish the walk.

Refuel at Highland Grill.

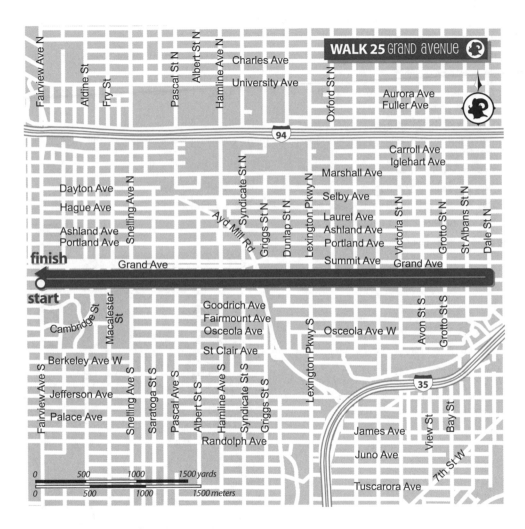

WALK 25 Grand Avenue

Fairview Ave N
Aldine St
Fry St
Pascal St N
Albert St N
Hamline Ave N
Charles Ave
University Ave
Oxford St N
Aurora Ave
Fuller Ave

94

Carroll Ave
Iglehart Ave

Dayton Ave
Hague Ave
Snelling Ave N
Syndicate St N
Marshall Ave
Selby Ave
Ayd Mill Rd
Griggs St N
Dunlap St N
Lexington Pkwy N
Laurel Ave
Ashland Ave
Portland Ave
Victoria St N
Grotto St N
St Albans St N
Dale St N

Ashland Ave
Portland Ave
Summit Ave

finish
Grand Ave
Grand Ave

start

Cambridge St
Macalester St
Goodrich Ave
Fairmount Ave
Osceola Ave
St Clair Ave
Avon St S
Grotto St S
Osceola Ave W

Berkeley Ave W
Lexington Pkwy S

Fairview Ave S
Jefferson Ave
Palace Ave
Snelling Ave S
Saratoga St S
Pascal Ave S
Albert St S
Hamline Ave S
Syndicate St S
Griggs St S

35

James Ave
View St
Bay St
Juno Ave
Randolph Ave
7th St W
Tuscarora Ave

0   500   1000   1500 yards
0   500   1000   1500 meters

25 Grand Avenue: Everybody Loves a Parade

BOUNDARIES: Grand Ave., Fairview Ave., Dale St.
HUDSON'S TWIN CITY STREET ATLAS **COORDINATES: Map 422, 2A, 3A, and 4A**
DISTANCE: Approx. 5 miles
DIFFICULTY: Easy
PARKING: Free parking on Grand Ave.
PUBLIC TRANSIT: Bus line 63

This walk follows the parade route of St. Paul's famous annual warm-weather event, Grand Old Day. On the first Sunday of June, pedestrians along Grand Ave. can watch entire worlds unfold down Grand Ave.—high school rock bands and professional Irish bands, jugglers and acrobats, mini petting zoos, inflatable rubber castles, rock climbing walls; you name it, and it's probably been at Grand Old Day at least once. The first Grand Old Day was held in 1973 in what was then considered to be a neighborhood suffering from urban blight; since then, the area has transformed itself into one of the most eclectic, upscale neighborhoods in St. Paul.

Dozens of shops and restaurants line this route. We're listing only our own favorites, with the hopes that you'll explore beyond these recommendations.

● Start at the corner of Fairview Ave. and Grand Ave., on the south side of the street, in front of Grandview Grill. This place is a local favorite for good reason, and during the Grand Old Day celebration it's nearly impossible to get a table here from 6 a.m. to closing.

● Go straight east down Grand Ave. and past Dog Days, which sells everything from cheap biscuits to fancy, upscale toys for your walking companion. Cross Wheeler and go straight. Cow Bella Gelato makes their specialty gelati and sorbets in-house, featuring a fantastic range of flavors, from strawberry to fig-and–goat cheese.

● Cross Cambridge St. and go straight. Shish Mediterranean Grill and Café has fantastic Middle Eastern food—including what is possibly the best falafel in the Twin Cities—as well as a great selection of coffee, teas, and desserts.

- Cross Macalester St. and keep going straight east. Most of this block is taken by the Macalester College campus, a liberal-arts college that's a focal point of the neighborhood.

  Cross the bridge and go straight to keep following Grand Ave. east. Below you is Ayd Mill Rd., an old service road built through the valley of what was once Cascade Creek, which was diverted many years ago to run almost exclusively underground.

  Cross Snelling Ave. On the left is Garrison Keillor's Common Good Books, a pretty good bookstore.

- Cross Dunlap St. and go straight. Bravo! Café & Bakery sells homemade, filled-on-the-spot cream puffs, mango and pineapple cakes, and other delectable desserts.

- Cross Victoria St. and go straight. If you're still hungry, you're in luck—on the corner is Café Latte, home of some of the most amazing cheesecakes, tortes, soups, pizzas, and sandwiches, and, of course, coffee in the area. Tavern on Grand is famous for its walleye—a plate of the lightly seasoned fish (a Minnesotan specialty) with a mug of the Tavern's chilled beer makes for a perfect lunch, any time of year.

- At Dale St., turn left and cross the street, and then immediately turn left again to walk down the other side of Grand Ave. In front of the Kirkland Apartments at 657 Grand stands an exceptional, hand-carved, life-size statue of a soldier sitting next to a child. The Dale Apartments (628 Grand Ave.) served as the secret hideout for the Barker-Karpis gang in December 1933 when they planned the kidnapping of financier Edward Bremer.

- Cross Victoria St., and you'll come to Victoria Crossing, an indoor mini-mall offering wonderful dining and shopping. The mall is much bigger than it looks on the outside—spacious walkways, potted plants, and a cobblestone-and-brick interior give the illusion that you're walking through an outdoor alleyway rather than the inside of a building. Some of the must-visit spots inside the mall include the Café Latte–owned Bread and Chocolate, which makes wonderful scones, cookies, and sandwiches; The Bead Monkey, which carries hundreds of bead and jewelry notions in every style; and 10,000 Villages, which carries fair-trade items from around the world. A couple of doors down from Victoria Crossing is the Red Balloon Bookshop, a notable independent children's bookstore that hosts readings by local and national children's authors, and even the occasional in-store petting zoo.

● Cross Hamline Ave. Just Truffles is a local confectionary that got its start in the lobby of the elegant St. Paul Hotel. It was featured on *The Oprah Winfrey Show* a few years ago as making the best chocolate truffles in the country, and many celebrities make it a habit to stop here for one of the specialty chocolates whenever they're in town.

● Cross Fairview Ave. to return to our starting point.

POINTS OF INTErest

Grandview Grill newgrandviewgrill.com, 1818 Grand Ave., St. Paul, MN 55105, 651-698-2346

Dog Days dogdaysinc.com, 1752 Grand Ave., St. Paul, MN 55105, 651-642-9663

Cow Bella Gelato cowbellagelato.com, 1700 Grand Ave., St. Paul, MN 55105, 651-340-0585

Shish Mediterranean Grill and Café shishcafe.net, 1668 Grand Ave., St. Paul, MN 55105, 651-690-2212

Macalester College macalester.edu, 1600 Grand Ave., St. Paul, MN 55105, 651-696-6000

Common Good Books commongoodbooks.com, 38 Snelling Ave. S., St. Paul, MN 55105, 651-225-8989

Bravo! Café & Bakery bravobakery.net, 1106 Grand Ave., St. Paul, MN 55105, 651-287-9118

Café Latte cafelatte.com, 850 Grand Ave., St. Paul, MN 55105, 651-224-5687

Tavern on Grand tavernongrand.com, 656 Grand Ave., St. Paul, MN 55105, 651-228-9030

Victoria Crossing 850 Grand Ave., St. Paul, MN 55105, 800-872-2657

Red Balloon Bookshop redballoonbookshop.com, 891 Grand Ave., St. Paul, MN 55105, 651-224-8320

Just Truffles justtruffles.com, 1363 Grand Ave., St. Paul, MN 55105, 651-690-0075

route summary

1. Start at the corner of Fairview Ave. and Grand Ave., on the south side of the street.
2. Go straight east down Grand Ave. until you get to Dale St.
3. Turn left and cross the street, and then immediately turn left again to walk down the other side of Grand Ave.
4. Go all the way west down Grand Ave. until you get back to Fairview Ave., right back where we started.

dog days

www.urbanimal.com

Natural Foo

Unique Pet
Products

Treat Fido to a biscuit at Dog Days.

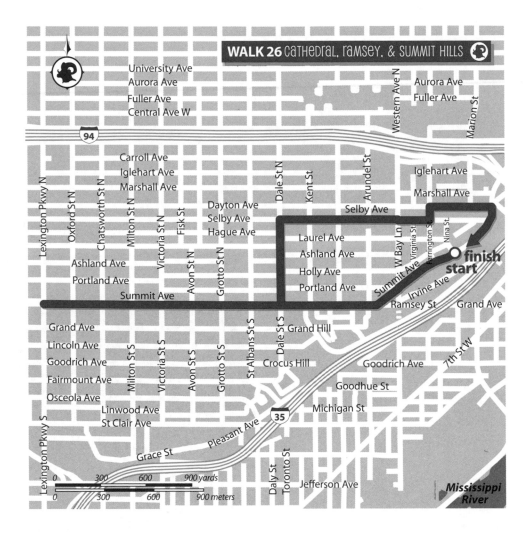

University Ave
Aurora Ave
Fuller Ave
Central Ave W

Aurora Ave
Fuller Ave

Western Ave N

Marion St

94

Carroll Ave
Iglehart Ave
Marshall Ave

Iglehart Ave

Marshall Ave

Dale St N

Kent St

Arundel St

Lexington Pkwy N

Oxford St N

Chatsworth St N

Milton St N

Victoria St N

Fisk St

Dayton Ave
Selby Ave
Hague Ave

Selby Ave

Nina St.

Ashland Ave
Portland Ave

Avon St N

Grotto St N

Laurel Ave
Ashland Ave
Holly Ave
Portland Ave

W Bay Ln

Virginia St

Farrington S

**finish
start**

Summit Ave

Summit Ave

Irvine Ave

Ramsey St

Grand Ave

Grand Ave
Lincoln Ave
Goodrich Ave
Fairmount Ave
Osceola Ave

Milton St S

Victoria St S

Avon St S

Grotto St S

St Albans St S

Dale St S

Grand Hill

Crocus Hill

Goodrich Ave

7th St W

Goodhue St

Michigan St

Linwood Ave
St Clair Ave

Lexington Pkwy S

Pleasant Ave

35

Grace St

Daly St

Toronto St

Jefferson Ave

*Mississippi
River*

0   300   600   900 yards
0   300   600   900 meters

Cathedral, Ramsey, & Summit Hills: Linking August Past with Dynamic Present

BOUNDARIES: Summit Ave., Lexington Pkwy. N., Dayton Ave.
HUDSON'S TWIN CITY STREET ATLAS **COORDINATES: Map 395, 5D; Map 422, 4A and 5A**
DISTANCE: Approx. 4¼ miles
DIFFICULTY: Moderate
PARKING: Free parking on Summit Ave.
PUBLIC TRANSIT: Bus line 63

The Cathedral, Ramsey, and Summit Hills—often referred to simply as the Hill District—was recognized by the National Register of Historic Places in 1976, and the area is acknowledged for some of the best-preserved Victorian homes in the U.S. However, it fell into hard times in the Depression years of the '30s. It did not recover until the late '60s, when urban pioneers purchased the homes, often for a pittance of their value, and restored them to their architectural glory. Located on the bluff above downtown St. Paul, the first mansions were built on Summit Hill in the 1850s, but many of the eclectic Victorian mansions were built in the 1880s. James J. Hill, the railroad-tycoon creator of the Great Northern Railway, built his massive red sandstone mansion in 1891.

Another landmark, the Cathedral of St. Paul, an architectural tribute to St. Peter's Basilica in Rome, was completed in 1915. Standing at 306½ feet above downtown, it looms over Cathedral Hill like an immense colossus of St. Cloud granite. In its shadow lies a substantial business district, as well as apartment and condo buildings on Selby Ave., a development legacy from when the long-gone streetcar system first connected the neighborhood to downtown in 1887. In the past 20 years, the Selby Ave. business district has become a hotbed for dining, drinking, and shopping. W. A. Frost & Company helped jump-start the area's renaissance in 1976, which continues even today.

● **Begin at the southeast corner of Summit Ave. and Nina St., and walk southwest down Summit Ave. to overlook downtown. This section of the street contains one notable home after another—even when the architecture is typical of a style, other distinctions are striking. On the left, the Stewart-Driscoll House (312 Summit Ave.), an Italian–style mansion, is the oldest house on Summit Ave. (1858). The next few homes, again on** the left, are early Cass Gilbert works. Gilbert later designed the Minnesota State Capitol, the U.S. Supreme Court, and the Woolworth Building in New York City. The William Lightner House (1893) at 318 Summit Ave. is an interesting combination of Richardsonian Romanesque and Classical Revival, while the William Lightner–George Young Double House (1888) at 322–24 Summit Ave. draws from Queen Anne and Renaissance Revival.

● Continue west on Summit Ave., passing a fine collection of eclectic Victorian homes. Straight ahead on the left, where Ramsey St. merges at the top of the hill and becomes Summit Ave., is Summit Park— stop for a panoramic view of St. Paul.

● After crossing Ramsey St., turn right on Summit Ave. Around the corner are a number of exceptional mansions. The University Club (420 Summit Ave.) is an excellent example of Tudor Revival architecture, built in 1913. Another impressive mansion is the limestone Italianate-style Burbank-Livingston-Griggs House (432 Summit Ave.) from 1863.

● Continue on Summit Ave. and notice the interesting combination of architectural styles. The Summit Terrace (587–601 Summit Ave.) brownstone row house was the residence of F. Scott Fitzgerald when he wrote his first novel, *This Side of Paradise*.

JaMES J. HILL: railroad TYCOON OF THE GILDED aGE

James J. Hill was an influential St. Paul businessman whose impact is still felt today. Hill was born of modest means in Ontario, Canada, in 1838. He started out in St. Paul working as a transportation clerk for riverboats on the levee of the Mississippi River. In 1878 Hill set out to make his fortune in the fledgling railroad industry, purchasing the nearly bankrupt St. Paul and Pacific Railroad with other financial partners. He quickly turned the railroad's finances around and added routes to Canada, the Rocky Mountains, and the West Coast. His business interests diversified into agriculture, shipping, mining, milling, finance, and banking. The companies he developed still exist today after mergers and consolidations as Burlington Northern Santa Fe Railroad and U.S. Bank. His legacy also continues in philanthropy—particularly the James J. Hill Reference Library in downtown St. Paul, a nonprofit, independent library founded in 1921.

● Continue west, crossing Dale St. After several blocks of lovely Victorians is the Tudor Revival–style Minnesota Governor's Residence (1006 Summit Ave.), which has served the state's chief executive since the late '60s.

● Turn right on Lexington Pkwy., and then immediately turn right on Summit Ave., where the corner is dominated by the immense and spectacular Italian and French Romanesque–inspired Saint Thomas More Catholic Church (1925).

● Continue along Summit Ave. in the opposite direction to cross Milton St., the location of William Mitchell College of Law, formerly St. Paul College of Law. The Warren E. Burger Library is named for the school's best-known alumnus, who was appointed by Richard Nixon in 1969 and served until 1986 as chief justice of the U.S. Supreme Court.

● Continue east into another impressive section of Summit Ave.'s mansion row. In 1908, St. Paul architect Clarence Johnston designed the colossal Samuel and Madeline Dittenhofer House (807 Summit Ave.), as well as 37 other homes on Summit Ave. He also created the William Elsinger House (701 Summit Ave.); it is immediately preceded by Cass Gilbert's design of the Jacob and Bettie Dittenhofer House (705 Summit Ave.).

● Cross Dale St. and turn left. Observe the variation in housing stock when walking away from Summit Ave. Just before Selby Ave. and on the right is the Muddy Pig, a neighborhood bar and restaurant offering some of the best in local and international craft beers.

● Turn right on Selby Ave. Kitty-corner is the Mississippi Market, a fantastic local co-op without a membership requirement. Continuing east on Selby Ave., dining options become more elegant, but one restaurant that is equally accessible is the Happy Gnome, a renovated fire station offering more than 40 beers on tap and 100 bottled beers, appetizers, and a full menu for alfresco dining in warm weather months. Dr. Chocolate's Chocolate Chateau is a chocolate shop for true chocolate lovers, featuring a wide range of gourmet chocolates from high-end, independent chocolatiers from all over the country.

● Continue east on Selby Ave., crossing Western Ave., where you have a stunning view of the Cathedral of Saint Paul to the east. Here you'll find several opportunities for fine dining. Located in the beautifully restored redbrick-and-sandstone Dacotah Building, W. A. Frost & Company serves upscale Mediterranean-influenced fare, with an emphasis on locally grown and organic ingredients. This neighborhood institution was mentioned in Jonathan Franzen's novel *Freedom.* Across the street is high-end Russian cuisine at Moscow on the Hill, where borscht, caviar, and pelmeni (meat dumplings) are served with an extensive selection of vodkas and wines to wash them down.

● Turn left on Virginia St. and then turn right on Selby Ave. at Boyd Park, named after Frank Boyd, who was instrumental in organizing local railroad porters. Across the street is Cass Gilbert's cute little Virginia Street Church (formerly Swedenborgian Church). This charmer was constructed in 1887 with clapboard, river stones, and shingles.

● Turn left on Farrington St., passing Boyd Park, and turn right on Dayton Ave. This area is loaded with restored Victorian apartments and condos.

● Descend the hill on Dayton Ave. to reach the colossal Cathedral of Saint Paul, which opened on Palm Sunday in 1915. Designed by Emmanuel Masqueray, the structure was inspired by St. Peter's Basilica in Rome but showcases St. Cloud (Minnesota) granite. It can seat 3,000 parishioners for Mass.

● Turn right on Summit Ave. and ascend the hill in the Victorian mansion row to finish the walk. On the left is the James J. Hill House, the great mansion built by the St. Paul railroad mogul for his 10 children. It is now owned and operated by the Minnesota Historical Society.

POINTS OF INTEREST

Summit Park tinyurl.com/summitparkmn, 185 Summit Ave., St. Paul, MN 55102, 651-632-5111

Minnesota Governor's Residence admin.state.mn.us/govres, 1006 Summit Ave., St. Paul, MN 55105, 651-201-3464

Saint Thomas More Catholic Church morecommunity.org, 1093 Summit Ave., St. Paul, MN 55105, 651-227-7669

William Mitchell College of Law wmitchell.edu, 875 Summit Ave., St. Paul, MN 55105, 651-227-9171

Muddy Pig muddypig.com, 162 Dale St., St. Paul, MN 55102, 651-254-1030

Mississippi Market msmarket.coop, 622 Selby Ave., St. Paul, MN 55104, 651-310-9499

Happy Gnome thehappygnome.com, 498 Selby Ave., St. Paul, MN 55102, 651-287-2018

Dr. Chocolate's Chocolate Chateau drchocolate.com, 579 Selby Ave., St. Paul, MN 55102, 651-379-3676

W. A. Frost & Company wafrost.com, 374 Selby Ave., St. Paul, MN 55102, 651-324-5715

Moscow on the Hill moscowonthehill.com, 371 Selby Ave., St. Paul, MN 55102, 651-291-1236

Boyd Park tinyurl.com/boydpark, 335 Selby Ave., St. Paul, MN 55102, 651-632-5111

Virginia Street Church virginiastreetchurch.org, 170 Virginia St., St. Paul, MN 55102, 651-224-4553

Cathedral of Saint Paul cathedralsaintpaul.org, 239 Selby Ave., St. Paul, MN 55102, 651-228-1766

James J. Hill House mnhs.org/places/sites/jjhh, 240 Summit Ave., St. Paul, MN 55102, 651-297-2555

route summary

1. Begin at the southeast corner of Summit Ave. and Nina St. and walk southwest down Summit Ave. to overlook downtown.
2. After crossing Ramsey St., turn right on Summit Ave.
3. Turn right on Lexington Pkwy. and then immediately turn right onto Summit Ave.
4. Cross Dale St. and turn left.
5. Turn right on Selby Ave.
6. Turn left on Virginia St. and turn right on Selby Ave. at Boyd Park.
7. Turn left on Farrington St., passing Boyd Park, and turn right on Dayton Ave.
8. Turn right on Summit Ave. and ascend the hill in the Victorian mansion row to finish the walk.

Stop in for a craft beer at The Muddy Pig.

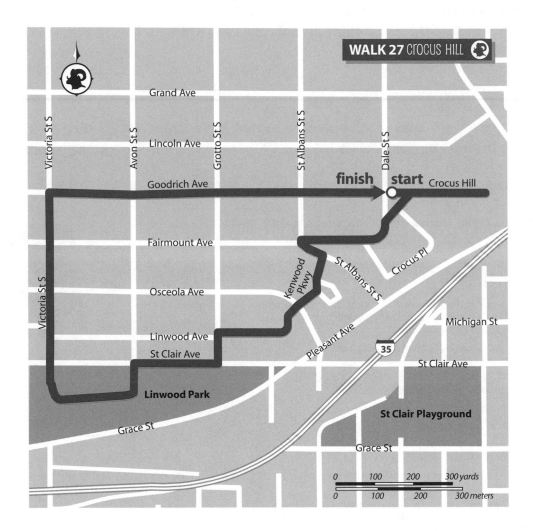

Grand Ave

Victoria St S

Avon St S

Lincoln Ave

Grotto St S

St Albans St S

Dale St S

Goodrich Ave

finish **start** Crocus Hill

Fairmount Ave

Kenwood Pkwy

St Albans St S

Crocus Pl

Osceola Ave

Linwood Ave

Pleasant Ave

St Clair Ave

Michigan St

35

St Clair Ave

Linwood Park

St Clair Playground

Grace St

Grace St

0   100   200   300 yards

0   100   200   300 meters

27 Crocus Hill: a glimpse into a decadent past

BOUNDARIES: **Grace St., Pleasant Ave., Victoria St. S., Goodrich Ave., Dale St. S., St. Albans St. S., Kenwood Pkwy.**

HUDSON'S TWIN CITY STREET ATLAS COORDINATES: **Map 422, 4A and 5A**

DISTANCE: **Approx. 2 miles**

DIFFICULTY: **Strenuous**

PARKING: **Parking on Goodrich Ave./Crocus Hill**

PUBLIC TRANSIT: **Bus line 67**

If you're into swank old mansions and the ritzy, glitzy days of St. Paul's past, then this is the walk for you. Crocus Hill, considered to be the newest section of the Hill District despite its 130-plus-year pedigree, is a remarkable neighborhood loaded with beautiful old estates listed on the National Historic Landmarks register. Throughout the summer, walking tours, garden tours, and home tours are often offered. The neighborhood features mansions that were built in the late 1800s, as well as a prime location just blocks away from Grand Ave.'s trendy shops and restaurants.

● **Start at Dale St. S. and Goodrich Ave.**

● **Walk toward Crocus Hill, as directed on the street sign.**

● **Go straight east on the left side of the street until you reach the end of the block. The Tudor Revival house at 15 Crocus Hill was built in 1922 and is listed on the National Register of Historic Places. The bronze statue at nearby Cochran Park, *Indian Hunter and His Dog,* was a gift to the city from the house's original owners, Mr. and Mrs. Arthur Savage. You can also see the silhouette of this statue on all the Crocus Hill banners along the neighborhood streets. The colossal redbrick Queen Anne at 4 Crocus Hill is the Rice-Merriam House. The original owner of this house was Edmund Rice Jr., son of Mayor/Representative/Senator Edmund Rice Sr. and nephew of Henry M. Rice, who worked to establish Minnesota's statehood and became Minnesota's first senator. The Georgian Revival house at 6 Crocus Hill is the T. L. Schurmeier House, built in 1903.**

- Cross the street and go back up Crocus Hill/Goodrich Ave., this time on the other side of the street.

- Follow the sidewalk as it continues around to the left where Fairmount Ave. intersects Dale St. S.

- At Crocus Pl., turn right to cross the street to the sidewalk.

- Turn left to follow Fairmount Ave. along the sidewalk to the left. The Georgian Revival brick house at 94 Crocus Pl. is the C. H. Biorn House, built in 1891. At 633 Fairmount Ave. is the large Queen Anne and Richardsonian Romanesque home of Minnesota's first popularly elected U.S. senator and Nobel Peace Prize recipient, Frank Billings Kellogg.

- Cross the street at St. Albans St. S. and turn left to cross Fairmount Ave. Turn left at the sidewalk and go straight to follow St. Albans St. S.

- Turn right at the corner to follow Kenwood Pkwy.

- Follow the brick wall and head uphill. At the corner by the ONE-WAY sign, turn right to go downhill.

- At the STOP sign at Osceola Ave. and Kenwood Pkwy., cross the brick cobblestone road and go straight.

- Follow the sidewalk up the hill and around to the right, following Linwood Ave. To your left are some amazing newer mansions at 703–725 Linwood Ave.

- Turn left on Grotto St. S. and pass the gorgeous yellow brick mansion at 226 Grotto, designed by Minnesotan architect John Wheeler in 1925.

- Walk to the end of the block and down the stairs that are set into the wall. From the stairs, you can see the old Schmidt Brewing Company factory just past the line of trees. Turn right at the bottom of the stairs to follow the massive retaining wall and St. Clair Ave. When you were walking along the streets at the top of the hill earlier, did you wonder where the people living in those majestic old mansions parked their cars? Down here, you'll have your answer: all along the wall to your right are modern garage doors—one or two under each house.

- Turn left at Avon St. S. to cross the street, and then go straight to follow the path into the park. To your left is a deep ravine full of old oak trees, while to your right is a huge field perfect for Frisbee throwing.

- Follow the path around to the overlook benches. Just below you is the I-35E freeway and train tracks. The bluffs below you are part of the Sam Morgan Prairie restoration site, named after longtime Crocus Hill resident and conservationist Samuel H. Morgan.

- Follow the path to the right to walk in front of the Linwood Community Recreation Center, where you'll find restrooms, drinking fountains, and a great baseball field just down the steps. Go up the short set of stairs in front of the building to your right and cross St. Clair Ave. at the crosswalk.

- Walk north to follow Victoria St. S. Cross Linwood Ave. and continue straight.

This is where we get into some of the best-preserved Victorians in the city. On the right side of the street, the house at 859 Osceola Ave., with the great columns and the cast iron balustrade, is listed on the National Register of Historic Places as part of the historic Hill District. On the left at 863 Osceola Ave. is the Charles Trudeau House, built in 1912. The Eastlake-style houses at 854–856 Fairmount Ave. used to be one big house: the William Garland House, built in 1890 and divided up into several residences in 1916. The neighboring house at 170 Victoria St. S. originally served as William Garland's carriage house.

- Turn right at Goodrich Ave. If you go straight from here instead of turning, you reach Victoria St. S. and Grand Ave. in about two blocks, where you can find great places to eat and drink (see Walk 25).

On the left side of the street at 851 Goodrich Ave. is the J. M. Gruber House, a Queen Anne built in 1915. Just down the street at 833 Goodrich Ave. is another gigantic Queen Anne, the Christopher C. Andrews House, built in 1882. At 825 Goodrich Ave. you'll find the John Weyerhaeuser House, built in 1888 for the son of Frederick Weyerhaeuser, the lumber baron whose name also graces Macalaster College's

Weyerhaeuser Chapel. At 796 Goodrich Ave. is the Georgian Revival–style manor and former home of Gregory McGuiggan, founder of the H. M. Smyth Printing Company; in the 1920s, he was the first printer west of Chicago to use lithography to produce books. At 781 Goodrich Ave. is the A. A. Doolittle House, a Georgian Revival designed and built in 1923 by Clarence H. Johnston Sr. At 748 Goodrich Ave. is the A. T. Koerner House, built in 1889; it's the former home of W. A. Frost, who in the 1900s ran a drugstore in the same location as the elegant restaurant that still bears his name. The Georgian Revival house at 725 Goodrich Ave. was originally the home of Armour & Company agent C. E. Gooch, who spent time in jail for selling margarine during the 1890s, back when the controversial substance was still illegal in Minnesota. The Shingle-style house at 634 Goodrich Ave. was designed by the state capitol's architect, Cass Gilbert, and built in 1890.

● At the end of the block is Dale St. S. and Goodrich Ave., where we started.

POINTS OF INTEREST

Cochran Park tinyurl.com/cochranpark, 375 Summit Ave., St. Paul, MN 55102, 651-632-5111

Sam Morgan Prairie summithillassociation.org, 860 St. Clair Ave., St. Paul, MN 55105, 651-222-1222

Linwood Community Recreation Center tinyurl.com/linwoodparkmn, 860 St. Clair Ave., St. Paul, MN 55105, 651-298-5660

ROUTE SUMMARY

1. Start at Dale St. S. and Goodrich Ave.
2. Walk toward Crocus Hill, as directed on the street sign.
3. Go straight east on the left side of the street until you reach the end of the block.
4. Cross the street and go back up Crocus Hill/Goodrich Ave., this time on the other side of the street.
5. Follow the sidewalk as it continues around to the left where Fairmount Ave. intersects with Dale St. S.
6. At Crocus Pl., turn right to cross the street to the sidewalk.
7. Turn left to follow Fairmount Ave. along the sidewalk to the left.
8. Cross the street at St. Albans St. S. and turn left to cross Fairmount Ave.

9. Follow the brick wall and head uphill.

10. At the corner by the ONE-WAY sign, turn right to head down the hill.

11. At the STOP sign at Osceola Ave. and Kenwood Pkwy., cross the brick cobblestone road and go straight.

12. Follow the sidewalk uphill and around to the right, following Linwood Ave.

13. Turn left on Grotto St. S.

14. Go to the end of the block and down the stairs that are set into the wall.

15. Turn right at the bottom of the stairs to follow the massive retaining wall along St. Clair Ave.

16. At Avon St. S., turn left to cross the street, and then go straight to follow the path into the park.

17. Follow the path to the right to walk in front of the Linwood Community Recreation Center.

18. Go up the short set of stairs in front of the building to your right and cross St. Clair Ave. at the crosswalk.

19. Go straight to follow Victoria St. S.

20. At Goodrich Ave., turn right and go straight to the finish at Dale St. S.

For in-depth tours of the historic Summit Hill houses

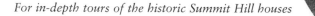

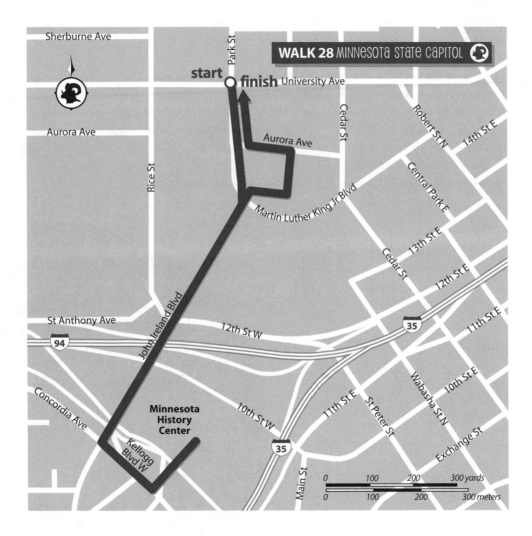

Sherburne Ave

Park St

start · finish · University Ave

Aurora Ave

Cedar St

Robert St N

14th St E

Central Park E

Rice St

Martin Luther King Jr Blvd

13th St E

Cedar St

12th St E

35

John Ireland Blvd

St Anthony Ave

12th St W

11th St E

94

Concordia Ave

Kellogg Blvd W

Minnesota History Center

10th St W

11th St E

St Peter St

Wabasha St N

10th St E

Exchange St

35

Main St

| 0 | 100 | 200 | 300 yards |
| 0 | 100 | 200 | 300 meters |

MINNESOTA STATE CAPITOL: SEAT OF GOVERNMENT OVERSEEING THE CAPITAL CITY

BOUNDARIES: **Kellogg Blvd. W., John Ireland Blvd., Rev. Dr. Martin Luther King Jr. Blvd., University Ave., Cedar St.**
HUDSON'S TWIN CITY STREET ATLAS **COORDINATES: Map 396, 1D**
DISTANCE: Approx. 1½ miles
DIFFICULTY: Moderate
PARKING: Metered parking available on University Ave.
PUBLIC TRANSIT: Bus line 16 and 50

The Minnesota State Capitol, including its adjoining mall, is an architectural masterpiece overlooking scenic downtown St. Paul. The building is situated between downtown and the working-class Frogtown neighborhood, but it is visible for miles because of its immense size. It is one of the state's most beloved architectural landmarks, and for good reason. The current building is the third capitol building in the state's history; its predecessors were destroyed by fire or deemed too small. It is the result of a statewide design competition that was awarded to 35-year-old St. Paul architect Cass Gilbert in 1895. The masterful, well-proportioned design—glimmering white marble in neoclassical style—belied the architect's youthful age. However, it went over budget and was not completed until 1905. Legislators complained that the capitol was an extravagant misuse of public funds, but the furor dissipated after it was finished. From the mall you're afforded incredible views of the building's scope, down to its details, including Daniel French and Edward Potter's *Quadriga* (1906)—the elegant horse sculptures at the base of the capitol's dome. Plus, don't forget the view of the capitol from the Minnesota History Center, where you can also catch an excellent exhibit on Cass Gilbert.

● Begin on University Ave. and proceed south on Rev. Dr. Martin Luther King Jr. Blvd., on the west side of the capitol. If the legislature is in session, politicians and lobbyists are in abundance across from the prosaic State Office Building (1932).

● Continue south, crossing the parking lot exit. On the left is a statue of Floyd B. Olson, the Farmer–Labor Party governor who guided the state during the Great Depression and New Deal, only to see his national political aspirations thwarted by terminal cancer in 1936.

● Turn right at the crosswalk on Rev. Dr. Martin Luther King Jr. Blvd., and head south on John Ireland Blvd. On the mall are numerous statues and memorials. *Roy Wilkins Memorial (Spiral of Justice)* honors the civil rights leader's 46 years of service to the NAACP.

● Cross Rice St./12th St. W. To the left is one of several great views of downtown St. Paul.

● Turn left on Kellogg Blvd. W. As you descend the hill, you'll come to another scenic vista.

● Turn left and follow the sidewalk to the entrance of the Minnesota History Center, home of the Minnesota Historical Society's research libraries, interactive and touring exhibits, and an auditorium for films and lectures. It is one of the state's oldest institutions, existing since Minnesota became a territory in 1849. Inside is Café Minnesota, an excellent place for coffee, soup, or an entire meal with a regional flair.

● After exploring the Minnesota Historical Society and its grounds, return to Kellogg Blvd.

● Turn right on Kellogg Blvd. and return up the incline named after Frank B. Kellogg, the state's first elected U.S. Senator (1916), and Secretary of State under President Calvin Coolidge. He received the Nobel Peace Prize for the Kellogg-Briand Peace Pact in 1928, when France and the United States, frustrated after the devastation of World War I, attempted to outlaw war through legislation and diplomacy—a utopian policy that was later criticized as politically naïve.

● Turn right on John Ireland Blvd., named after the third bishop and first archbishop (1888) of the Roman Catholic Archdiocese of St. Paul and Minneapolis.

● After crossing Rice St./12th St. W., continue straight briefly before turning right on the first sidewalk. Absorb the grandeur of the mall and the capitol to the left on the horizon. As you approach the Veterans Service Building at the center of the mall, you'll pass numerous war memorials.

Nearby & Notable

The Frogtown neighborhood, part of which was recently rechristened Little Mekong (the five blocks between Galtier Ave. and MacKuban Ave.), is located east of the Minnesota State Capitol. This area is one of the Twin Cities' best areas for delicious, adventurous, and inexpensive dining. University Ave. is lined with a diverse array of ethnic cuisines, especially Southeast Asian, with excellent Vietnamese, Thai, Cambodian, Hmong, and Chinese restaurants for all tastes and pocketbooks. Que Nha features spring rolls, stir-fries, hot pots, *pho* (beef noodle soup), and Vietnamese items unavailable anywhere else in the Twin Cities in a comfortable, casual setting. Ngon Bistro offers Vietnamese food in a white-tablecloth atmosphere—outstanding versions of Asian fusion fare are paired with homey standards such as egg roll salad, *pho*, and a quaffable wine list. Little Szechuan is another excellent dining choice, specializing in Chengdu (the capital of Szechuan) Chinese cuisine such as *dan dan* noodles, *ma po* tofu, and authentic versions of kung pao dishes. Cheng Heng Restaurant serves superb, one-of-a-kind Cambodian fare in a relaxed, genuinely "mom, pop, and baby" atmosphere. The menu includes standard Asian items such as fried rice, but the real standouts are the authentic dishes—*chha* mussels, mussels in black bean sauce, and *banh cheo*, a rice-flour crepe served with pork, shrimp, raw vegetables, and fish sauce. And if that isn't yummy and cheap enough, then head for the astonishing values inside 88 Oriental Foods deli: a steam table of chicken, beef, and pork stir-fries, soups, and fresh spring rolls at mind-bogglingly low prices, great for a picnic.

Que Nha 849 University Ave. W., St. Paul, MN 55104, 651-290-8552

Ngon Bistro ngonbistro.com, 799 University Ave. W., St. Paul, MN 55104, 651-222-3301

Little Szechuan littleszechuan.com, 422 University Ave. W., St. Paul, MN 55103, 651-222-1333

Cheng Heng Restaurant 448 University Ave. W., St. Paul, MN 55103, 651-222-5577

88 Oriental Foods 291 University Ave. W., St. Paul, MN 55103, 651-209-8388

- At the Veterans Service Building (1954), turn left on one of the two sidewalks that bisect the building and the mall. This symmetrical modern building is situated directly south of the capitol on the mall.

- Continue on the parallel sidewalks, passing several Minnesota war memorials. The first is the World War II Memorial, a recent addition in 2007. The oval memorial features 10 glass panels that detail the sacrifices of Minnesotans—more than 320,000 served, 1,250 were prisoners of war, and 6,000 died. Up ahead on the left is the Minnesota Vietnam Veterans Memorial (1992), where the names of the Minnesotans killed or missing in action are written in granite.

- Continue on the mall and carefully cross Rev. Dr. Martin Luther King Jr. Blvd. In spring, summer, and early fall, the flower beds here are especially colorful.

- Walk up the stairs of the capitol and, time permitting, visit its interior and join the insightful Minnesota Historical Society tour.

- If you are not going inside the capitol, turn left.

- Turn right on Rev. Dr. Martin Luther King Jr. Blvd. and follow it to University Ave. to finish the walk.

POINTS OF INTEREST

Minnesota State Capitol mnhs.org/places/sites/msc, 75 Rev. Dr. Martin Luther King Jr. Blvd., St. Paul, MN 55155, 651-296-2881

Minnesota History Center mnhs.org, 345 Kellogg Blvd. W., St. Paul, MN 55102, 651-259-3900

Minnesota Vietnam Veterans Memorial mvvm.org, 20 12th St. W., St. Paul, MN 55155, 651-777-0686

route summary

1. Begin on University Ave. and proceed south on Rev. Dr. Martin Luther King Jr. Blvd.

2. Continue forward, crossing the parking lot exit.

3. At the crosswalk on Rev. Dr. Martin Luther King Jr. Blvd., turn right and then head south on John Ireland Blvd.

4. Turn left on Kellogg Blvd. W.

5. Turn left, following the sidewalk to the entrance of the Minnesota History Center.

6. After enjoying the Minnesota Historical Society and its grounds, return to Kellogg Blvd.

7. Turn right on Kellogg Blvd. and return up the incline.

8. Turn right on John Ireland Blvd.

9. After crossing Rice St., continue straight briefly before turning right on the first sidewalk.

10. At the Veterans Service Building at the center of the mall, turn left on one of the two sidewalks that bisect the building and the mall.

11. Continue on the parallel sidewalks.

12. Continue on the mall and carefully cross Rev. Dr. Martin Luther King Jr. Blvd.

13. Walk up the stairs of the capitol. If you are not going inside the capitol, turn left.

14. Turn right on Rev. Dr. Martin Luther King Jr. Blvd. to University Ave. and finish the walk.

Charles Lindberg Memorial

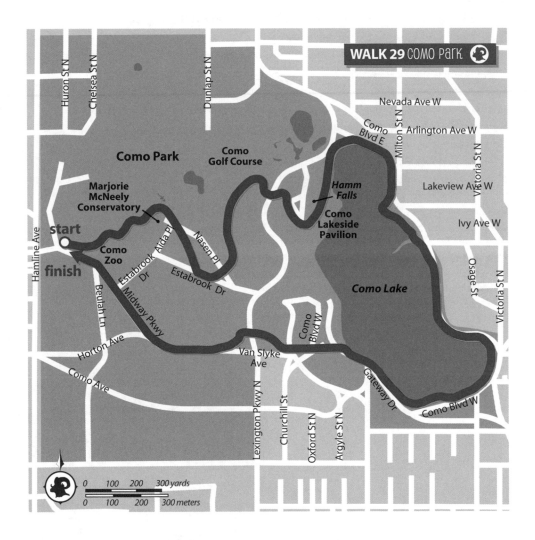

Como Park

Como Golf Course

Marjorie
McNeely
Conservatory

Hamm
Falls

Como
Lakeside
Pavilion

Hamline Ave

start

finish

Como
Zoo

Estabrook

Arda Pl

Dr

Nasen Pl

Estabrook Dr

Como Lake

Como
Blvd E

Milton St N

Nevada Ave W

Arlington Ave W

Victoria St N

Lakeview Ave W

Ivy Ave W

Osage St

Victoria St N

Beulah Ln

Midway Pkwy

Horton Ave

Como Ave

Van Slyke
Ave

Como
Blvd W

Gateway Dr

Como Blvd W

Lexington Pkwy N

Churchill St

Oxford St N

Argyle St N

Huron St N

Chelsea St N

Dunlap St N

0   100   200   300 yards
0   100   200   300 meters

29 COMO Park: ST. Paul's urBan retreat

BOUNDARIES: Como Ave., Hamline Ave., Arlington Ave. W., Como Blvd. E., Como Blvd. W.
HUDSON'S TWIN CITY STREET ATLAS **COORDINATES:** Map 395, 3B and 4B
DISTANCE: Approx. 2¾ miles
DIFFICULTY: Moderate
PARKING: Como Zoo parking lot; free parking on Horton Ave. and Midway Pkwy.
PUBLIC TRANSIT: Bus lines 3 and 61

Since 1887, Como Park has been a favorite retreat for St. Paul residents and visitors alike. Within its 300-plus acres of parkland are hiking trails, historic bridges and monuments, a free zoo, a restored wooden carousel, an amazing glass-enclosed conservatory, a Japanese garden, multiple butterfly and wildflower gardens, picnic grounds, baseball fields, an amusement park, a pavilion that offers live music during the summer, and, of course, Como Lake. Since the park's opening, the grounds have been worked by some of the finest gardeners in the world, starting in the early 1900s with Itchikawa, landscape gardener for the Mikado of Japan.

● In Como Park, start at the front of historic Cafesjian's Carousel. Look for the smallest of the three buildings in the Como Zoo lot—it's the brown wooden one with the horse weather vane mounted on the top, playing loud calliope music during the spring, summer, and early fall months.

● Follow the sidewalk along the carousel and take a right at the sidewalk fork.

● Take your first left to head toward the zoo and conservatory—the two impossible-to-miss large glass buildings at the end of the lot. The building to your right with the angular glass skylights is the entrance to Como Zoo, one of the oldest free zoos in the country. The amazing arabesque glass building ahead of you is the Marjorie McNeely Conservatory, whose gardens got their official start in 1915, when a group of ambitious gardeners planted seeds to grow the first fig and orange trees in the conservatory.

● Go straight down the path toward the conservatory. All along this walk are native flowers and grasses, as well as exotic flowers and plants, in planters. As you approach the conservatory, take a moment to stop and smell the roses—or lilies, or freesias, or

whatever else is in bloom in the conservatory's Sunken Garden. The fragrance of the flowers inside is so powerful that you can smell them through the glass.

- Take a right to go past the original entrance of the conservatory, now closed.

- Go straight past the conservatory steps and turn right to cross Aida Pl. Follow the path through the Monarch Waystation and the Enchanted Garden, where butterfly-attracting plants are grown.

- Follow the path to your right to walk beside the Frog Pond, built on the site of the park's first Japanese Garden. Head down to the stairs and go straight.

- Turn right at the fork and make an immediate left. Follow the path to cross the street and pick it up on the other side. Old oak trees are scattered throughout the many picnic areas.

- Cross the parking lot and stay on the path. On your left are the Como Golf Course and Cross Country Ski Area—which may sound like a strange combination if you're here in the summer, but spend one winter here and you'll realize what a brilliant idea this multiuse space is.

- Follow the serpentine path through the park and stay to the left when you come to the first fork. This takes you past a picturesque pond and over the pedestrian bridge that crosses Lexington Pkwy. N. Up ahead and to your right is Como Lake. The entire park was built with the lake as its focal point, and throughout its history the kidney-shaped lake has been a magnet for bird-watchers, boaters, fishermen, and those out for a romantic stroll. On a more ominous note, when a survey team temporarily drained the lake back in 1923 they found a weighted-down box of human bones. The bones were once believed to belong to the late James-Younger Gang member Charlie Pitts, whose body had never been recovered after Jesse James & Co. were gunned down in Northfield, Minnesota. DNA evidence recently proved that the skeleton comes from a yet-identified individual that may have died as early as the 1700s.

- Turn right after crossing the bridge and follow the path around to the left. The big building up ahead is the Como Lakeside Pavilion.

- Take your first left to go up to the beautiful, albeit artificial, Hamm Memorial Water Falls. If it's a hot day, this is a wonderful place to stop and cool down.

- Head straight and take the first right to go down the hill toward the pavilion. In the summer, you can catch free concerts in the open-air porch out back, including chamber music and performances by local gamelan groups. Inside the building, Black Bear Crossings on the Lake is a great place to pick up soups, sandwiches, pastries, and drinks.

- Cross the driveway and keep going straight. Take your first left to follow the lakeshore.

  On both sides of the path are native wildflowers and grasses, while on any given summer day egrets, herons, ducks, and Canada geese can be seen on the water.

- Stay on the right path (the official pedestrian path) to follow the curve of the lake. Look closely at the cattail and reed thickets you're passing—they're a great place to spot nesting geese and ducks, as well as their hatchlings. On your left is Como Blvd. E., which has an abundance of benches if you need to take a break.

- When you reach the first parking lot, take the right path around the lot. Then turn left on the gravel path. The rustic, rock-lined pathway takes you just shy of shore level, where you can get a closer look at the wetland flora and fauna. In the spring, this path can get a little swampy, but a little mud on your shoes is well worth the view.

Cafesjian's Carousel

- Turn right when you reach asphalt again. On your left is a small pocket of natural wetland that serves as yet another nesting place for waterfowl.

- Follow the path uphill to your left, and go straight to follow the contour of the lake. The boxes you see mounted on posts in the lake are for wood duck nests. In the wild, wood ducks make their nests up in the trees, and the chicks jump from great heights to bounce on the ground before searching out the nearest body of water. The boxes are a pleasant compromise for city-dwelling wood ducks that must fight squirrels for nesting rights in the trees.

- At the next fork, stay on the right path to follow the lake. If you enjoy fishing, the large wooden dock to your right is the place to do it. Nonresidents and residents alike can order a fishing license from the Minnesota Department of Natural Resources (dnr.state.mn.us), which entitles you to fish not only here but also at dozens of other lakes throughout the metro area.

- Go straight past the dock and parking lot, and continue following the lakeshore. On your right are old stands of cottonwoods and willows, home to local roosting birds as well as kingfishers and swallows.

- At the next fork, take the left path and make a left turn toward the street.

- Cross Como Blvd. W. and go straight and to your left to follow Horton Ave. Follow the sidewalk along the stone retaining wall.

- Cross Churchill St. and go straight.

- Just before you get to Lexington Pkwy. N., turn right to head down the path. From here, you can get a closer look at the Historic Streetcar Station. The station has limited visiting hours, but you can walk around the grounds to view the exterior and the former streetcar bridge just behind it.

- Take the left fork and follow the path straight, heading west.

- Take your first left to follow the path under the bridge. From here, you can get a good picture of where the old streetcar line used to run.

- Go straight and follow the path to the left.

- At the fork, take the left path and continue following it to the right.

- Turn right at the fork and go straight, heading northwest. On your right is a great big picnic area; the large pavilion up ahead has restrooms, drinking fountains, and additional picnic tables.

- Go straight across the parking lot entrance, and follow the path along Horton Ave.

- At Midway Pkwy., turn right.

- Go straight to cross the parking lot entrance, and go straight past the fork. Follow the path up the hill and through the woods.

- At the street crossing, look ahead and to the right. The big brown building with the horse weather vane on top is Cafesjian's Carousel, which is where we started.

POINTS OF INTEREST

Cafesjian's Carousel ourfaircarousel.org, 1245 Midway Pkwy., St. Paul, MN 55103, 651-489-4628

Como Park Zoo and Conservatory comozooconservatory.org, 1360 Lexington Pkwy. N., St. Paul, MN 55103, 651-487-8200

Como Golf Course and Cross Country Ski Area tinyurl.com/comogolf or tinyurl.com/comoski, 1431 Lexington Pkwy. N., St. Paul, MN 55103, 651-488-9673

Como Lakeside Pavilion tinyurl.com/comopavilion, 1360 Lexington Pkwy. N., St. Paul, MN 55103, 651-488-4920

Historic Streetcar Station tinyurl.com/historicstreetcar, 1224 Lexington Pkwy. N., St. Paul, MN 55103, 651-632-5111

route summary

1. Start at Cafesjian's Carousel. Follow the sidewalk along the carousel and take a right at the sidewalk fork.

2. Take your first left to head toward the Como Park Zoo and Conservatory.

3. Go straight toward the Marjorie McNeely Conservatory.

4. Take a right to pass the original entrance of the conservatory.

5. Go straight past the conservatory steps, turn right to cross Aida Pl., and head straight down the path.

6. Follow the path to your right.

7. Go down the stairs and straight.

8. Turn right at the fork and make an immediate left.

9. Cross the street and follow the path; cross the parking lot and stay on the path.

10. Stay on the left path when you come to the first fork. Cross the bridge.

11. Turn right after crossing the bridge, and follow the path around to the left.

12. Take your first left to Hamm Memorial Water Falls.

13. Head straight and take the first right to head downhill.

14. Cross the driveway and take your first left.

15. Stay to the right and go around the lake.

16. Just past the fishing dock and the parking lot, take the left fork.

17. Turn left toward the street. Cross Como Blvd. W. and go straight and to your left to follow Horton Ave.

18. Just before you get to Lexington Pkwy. N., turn right onto the walking path.

19. Take your first left to follow the path under the bridge. Go straight and follow the path to the right.

20. At the fork, take the left path and follow it to the right.

21. Turn right at the next fork and go straight.

22. Turn right at Midway Pkwy.

23. Go straight to cross the parking lot entrance and go straight past the fork.

24. At the street crossing, look ahead and to the right to see Cafesjian's Carousel and finish the walk.

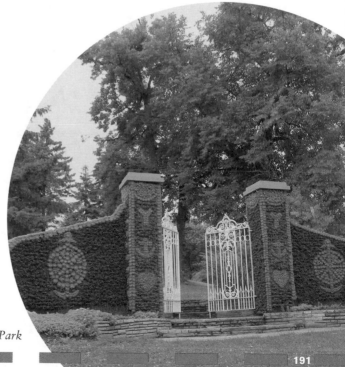

Gates Ajar floral display at Como Park

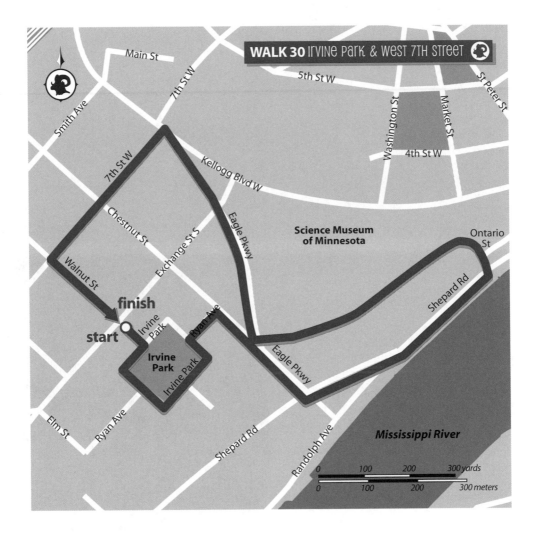

Main St

5th St W

7th St W

St Peter St

Smith Ave

7th St W

Kellogg Blvd W

Washington St

Market St

4th St W

Chestnut St

Eagle Pkwy

Science Museum
of Minnesota

Ontario
St

Exchange St S

Walnut St

Shepard Rd

finish

Ryan Ave

start

Irvine
Park

Eagle Pkwy

Irvine
Park

Irvine Park

Elm St

Ryan Ave

Shepard Rd

Randolph Ave

Mississippi River

| 0 | 100 | 200 | 300 yards |

| 0 | 100 | 200 | 300 meters |

30 Irvine Park & West 7th Street: Where the Oldest Neighborhood Meets the Newest Place to Play

BOUNDARIES: Shepard Rd., 7th St. W., Kellogg Blvd. W., Irvine Park
HUDSON'S TWIN CITY STREET ATLAS **COORDINATES:** Map 396, 1D; Map 423, 1A
DISTANCE: Approx. 1½ miles
DIFFICULTY: Moderate
PARKING: Limited 2-hour parking on Exchange St.
PUBLIC TRANSIT: Bus lines 3, 21, and 54

This walk juxtaposes St. Paul's oldest surviving neighborhood, Irvine Park, with the newest hot spot where St. Paul goes to party, West 7th St. Historically, the West 7th St. neighborhood was a hardscrabble, working-class, and close-knit community largely from two villages in southern Italy. The Italian immigrants made the most of the often-flooded Upper Levee Flats, later known as Little Italy. They were relocated by the city after 1960—Cossetta is one of the surviving businesses that moved up the hill from the levee, where Shepard Rd. and upscale condos are now located. Since Xcel Energy Center opened in 2000, the area has transformed into a bustling business district filled with restaurants and bars that are popular venues for celebrating after Minnesota Wild hockey games, concerts, conventions, and events.

In contrast, Irvine Park provides several examples of the state's history and fine architecture in a neighborhood that has been on the National Register of Historic Places since 1973. Plotted in 1849, the homes comprise a collection of types—restorations, those moved to the site, and recent in-fill construction. Enjoy the historic homes, and then sit down for a nosh and a drink, or an elegant meal and a bottle of wine.

● Begin at the corner of Walnut St. and Exchange St. S. and walk down Walnut St. On the right is Forepaugh's Restaurant, serving upscale continental cuisine in an immense three-story Victorian mansion with mansard roof (1870). It was once the home of a prominent dry-goods seller, Joseph Forepaugh, his wife, and two daughters. Shortly after moving in, he was caught having an affair with their maid, Molly, who soon after committed suicide. Today, the house is said to be haunted by entities of Molly and Joseph, who regularly appear as apparitions, turn the lights on and off, and make strange noises.

● Cross the intersection at Irvine Park and turn right on the sidewalk in the beautiful urban park, which started as a grazing area for horses in 1849 but has since been modified to its present splendor.

● At the corner of the park, turn left. Across the street are several historic homes. On the corner is the only Gothic Revival home in the neighborhood, the Jay and Henry Knox House (26 Irvine Park). Another beauty is the Parker-Marshall House (30 Irvine Park), built in 1852. It was at one time the home of William Marshall, who served as governor of Minnesota 1866–1870. The house has been moved several times—in both cases, only a few addresses down from 35 Irvine Park—as were several other homes in the area, including the Federal-style Simpson-Wood House, which was moved to 32 Irvine Park from nearby Sherman St.

● Cross Ryan Ave. and continue following the sidewalk in the park. Across the street is the Murray-Lanpher House (35 Irvine Park), an enormous Queen Anne from 1886. The Wagner-Marty House (38 Irvine Park) is a Greek Revival–style mansion that began its life in the 1850s in suburban Woodbury and now sits on the site of at least three previous homes.

● Turn left on Irvine Park. Among the many striking mansions on Walnut St., the classical grandeur of the Wright-Pendergast House (233 Walnut St.) stands out. The house was originally constructed in Greek Revival–style in 1851 but was substantially modified in 1907 with the addition of an immense neoclassical portico and Ionic pediment. On the corner is the Italianate John McDonald House (56 Irvine Park), constructed in 1873 and now turned into condominiums.

● Turn left on Irvine Park. Across the street is the Dr. Justus Ohage House (59 Irvine Park). The Romanesque Revival mansion was built in 1889 for the man responsible for creating St. Paul's public health system.

- Turn right on Ryan Ave. Constructed in 1851, the Humphrey-Willis House (240 Ryan Ave.) is unusual for the neighborhood because of its cottage size, but it is quite elegant in its symmetrical Georgian style. Next door, the Charles Symonds House (234 Ryan Ave.)—a simple structure built in 1850—is the oldest in St. Paul.

- Turn right on the one-way street that intersects with Eagle Pkwy. up the hill. Just before the railroad tracks is the Armstrong-Quinlan House, a double house that was built in 1886 as a rental property and later used as a nursing home. It was originally located on 5th St. in a vast parking lot across from the Xcel Energy Center, where it sat vacant for years. After countless studies and plans for its renovation, it was moved in 2001 for $2 million to its current site and converted to condos.

- Go straight ahead, heading southeast, and cross Shepard Rd.

- Turn left on Shepard Rd. on the path along the Mississippi River. From here, several paths lead to the water, park benches, and sculptures.

- Turn left on Ontario St., carefully crossing the railroad tracks, and follow the sidewalk along the perimeter of the Science Museum's Big Back Yard.

- Ascend the steps to the left until you reach the first level; then continue straight ahead. Above is the Science Museum of Minnesota, founded in 1907, though in a different location. The 370,000-square-foot building, including one temporary gallery and five permanent galleries, was opened in 1999 on this beautiful site overlooking the Mississippi River. Inside the museum,

Irvine Park fountain

alexander ramsey: Pioneer Politician

Alexander Ramsey was the first great politician in Minnesota—his impact is still felt today in the state's borders and in his namesake county that's home to the state capital. Like most early political and business leaders, his origins were outside the state; he arrived from Pennsylvania after President Zachary Taylor named him territorial governor. Ramsey was a Whig, and later a nascent Republican, in a territory dominated by Democrats. His early career as a politician in Minnesota was controversial, at best. His appointment by Washington, D. C. to negotiate with the Dakota Indians culminated in the treaties of 1851, which ceded vast lands to the area that became Minnesota for minimal money. This resentment, in part, led to the Dakota Conflict of 1862. Later, as a United States senator voicing a strong belief in manifest destiny, he called for annexing Rupert's Land, fur trade areas in central and western Canada. However, after the Civil War and in the era of the Reconstruction, there was little enthusiasm for pursuing his expansionist interests, and the state's original 1858 border remained.

The Minnesota Historical Society focuses on another side of Ramsey—his family life in the 1870s, during St. Paul's Victorian era. His home in the Irvine Park neighborhood includes exquisite marble furnaces and walnut woodwork, as well as more than 14,000 original furnishings.

the U.S. Department of the Interior runs the helpful Mississippi National River and Recreation Center.

- Cross the metal bridge. The Big Back Yard has combined a selection of native Minnesota trees, flowers, and grasses. Numerous markers provide explanation on the flora and its relationship to various natural biomes in the state and region.

- Follow the path as it veers right at the intersection after passing the Science House, a resource center for students and teachers that was constructed with state-of-the-art environmental technology.

- Follow the sidewalk on the outside perimeter of the park closest to the Science Museum.

- Cross Eagle Pkwy. and then turn right to cross Chestnut St. On the corner is *Charlie Andiamo Americano*—a sculpted tribute to St. Paul-born-and-raised *Peanuts* cartoonist Charles Schulz, and to the families who settled the Upper Levee. Up the steep hill is the Xcel Energy Center (or "the X"), which was completed in 2000. Home of the National Hockey League's Minnesota Wild, the building also hosts countless concerts and conventions, including the 2008 Republican National Convention. There's additional event space in the adjoining River Centre and Roy Wilkins Auditorium, the cozier venue named in honor of the great civil rights leader.

- Continue straight across 7th St. W. and immediately turn left to follow 7th St. W. This is the West 7th Street business district, where St. Paul celebrates after sporting events at the nearby Xcel Energy Center. On the right is The Liffey Irish Pub—this drinking establishment is the real McCoy, where a properly poured Guinness can be quaffed with appetizers or dinner on a comely terrace in warm weather. Just ahead is Cossetta's Italian Market and Pizzeria—as it advertises, "a taste of the levee"—where St. Paul's first Italian community was located and later forcibly relocated when the levee was declared unsafe for habitation. The recently renovated and expanded restaurant has the best old-school Little Italy–style cuisine in colossal proportions. Grab a workman-size slab of pizza and appreciate the wall-to-wall photos from the heyday of the levee. Upstairs is its upscale restaurant, Louis Ristorante & Bar.

- Cross Chestnut St. On the right is Patrick McGovern's Pub and Restaurant, a charming Irish bar for more than 20 years. Across the street is Tom Reid's Hockey City Pub—named after the former Minnesota North Star hockey player and announcer—a favorite hangout for watching hockey games on the big-screen televisions and for drinking cheap beer.

- After crossing Walnut St., turn left to cross 7th St. W., and continue on Walnut St. toward the Irvine Park neighborhood.

- Turn right on Exchange St. S. to finish the walk. At 265 Exchange St. S. is the Alexander Ramsey House, a lovely French Second Empire mansion built in 1872 for Minnesota's first territorial governor and second state governor.

POINTS OF INTEREST

Forepaugh's Restaurant forepaughs.com, 276 Exchange St. S., St. Paul, MN 55102, 651-224-5606

Irvine Park tinyurl.com/irvineparkmn, 251 Walnut St., St. Paul, MN 55102, 651-632-5111

Science Museum of Minnesota smm.org, 120 Kellogg Blvd. W., St. Paul, MN 55102, 651-221-9444

Mississippi National River and Recreation Area nps.gov/miss, 120 Kellogg Blvd. W., St. Paul, MN 55102, 651-292-0200

Xcel Energy Center xcelenergycenter.com, 175 Kellogg Blvd. W., St. Paul, MN 55102, 651-265-4800

Minnesota Wild Hockey Club wild.nhl.com, 317 Washington St., St. Paul, MN 55102, 651-602-6000

The Liffey Irish Pub theliffey.com, 175 7th St. W., St. Paul, MN 55102, 651-556-1420

Cossetta's Italian Market and Pizzeria/Louis Ristorante & Bar cossettas.com, 211 7th St. W., St. Paul, MN 55102, 651-222-3476

Patrick McGovern's Pub and Restaurant patmcgoverns.com, 225 7th St. W., St. Paul, MN 55102, 651-224-5821

Tom Reid's Hockey City Pub tomreidshockeycitypub.com, 258 7th St. W., St. Paul, MN 55102, 651-292-9916

Alexander Ramsey House mnhs.org/places/sites/arh, 265 Exchange St. S., St. Paul, MN 55102, 651-296-8760

ROUTE SUMMARY

1. Begin at the corner of Walnut St. and Exchange St. S. and walk down Walnut St.
2. Cross the intersection at Irvine Park, and turn right on the sidewalk.
3. Turn left at the corner of the park.
4. Turn left on Irvine Park.
5. Turn right on Ryan Ave.
6. Turn right on Eagle Pkwy.

7. Go straight ahead, heading southeast, and cross Shepard Rd.

8. Turn left on Shepard Rd.

9. Turn left on Ontario St.

10. Ascend the steps to the left until you reach the first level, and continue straight ahead.

11. Cross the metal bridge.

12. After passing the Science House, follow the path as it veers to the right at the intersection.

13. Follow the sidewalk on the outside perimeter closest to the Science Museum.

14. Cross Eagle Pkwy., and then turn right to cross Chestnut St.

15. Continue straight across 7th St. W. and immediately turn left to follow 7th St. W.

16. After crossing Walnut St., turn left to cross 7th St. W. and continue on Walnut St. toward the Irvine Park neighborhood.

17. Turn right on Exchange St. S. to finish the walk.

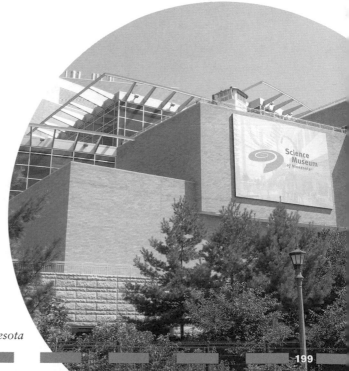

Science Museum of Minnesota

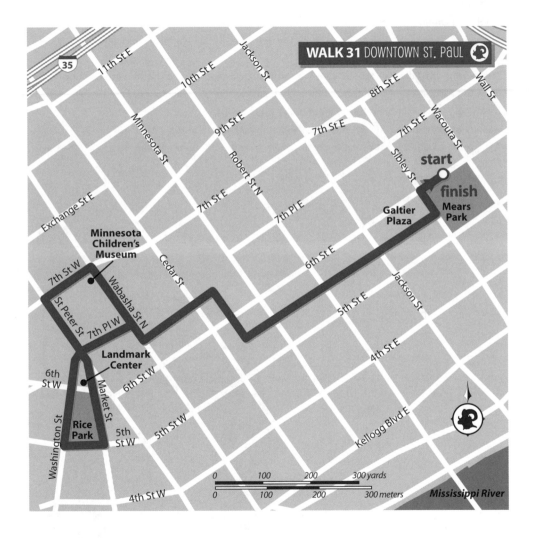

I-35

11th St E
10th St E
Jackson St
8th St E
Wall St
9th St E
7th St E
7th St E
Wacouta St
Minnesota St
Robert St N
7th Pl E
Sibley St
start
finish
Galtier Plaza
Mears Park
Exchange St E
7th St E
Cedar St
6th St E
Minnesota Children's Museum
7th W St
Wabasha St N
7th Pl W
St Peter St
5th St E
Jackson St
Landmark Center
6th St W
4th St E
6th St W
Market St
Kellogg Blvd E
Rice Park
5th St W
5th St W
Washington St
4th St W

0   100   200   300 yards
0   100   200   300 meters

Mississippi River

BOUNDARIES: 5th St. W., Washington St., 7th St. W., Wacouta St.
HUDSON'S TWIN CITY STREET ATLAS **COORDINATES: Map 396, 1D**
DISTANCE: Approx. 2 miles
DIFFICULTY: Easy
PARKING: 2-hour metered parking near Mears Park, on 5th St., 6th St., and Wacouta St.
PUBLIC TRANSIT: Numerous bus lines to Mears Park

Former Minnesota Governor Jesse Ventura once caused a near scandal by stating on the *Late Show with David Letterman* that St. Paul's streets were laid out by drunk Irishmen—a claim that car-driving visitors to the area have been more than happy to agree with. However, we think that the following St. Paul walk, starting at Mears Park and looping past Rice Park, might reveal a little bit of the genius in the madness. The angles of the streets and sidewalks give pedestrians the best possible view of the architecture, from the ornate buildings in Lowertown to the historic cultural centers that encircle Rice Park. In the winter, this area comes alive with Winter Carnival events, from subzero parades to sparkling ice sculptures; during the rest of the year, the streets are lined with flowers and perfectly manicured trees.

● Start at Mears Park, at the corner of 6th St. E. and Sibley St. Cross Sibley St. going southwest and turn left at Sibley to get to the Galtier Plaza entrance on Sibley St. across from Mears Park.

● Enter Galtier Plaza, named after Father Lucien Galtier, the Catholic priest who, in 1841, changed the name of the small settlement of Pig's Eye to Saint Paul's Landing, which was later shortened to St. Paul.

● Take the escalator up to the second floor and then turn right to go around the top of the escalator and head straight down the hall. As you're walking, you'll see the old Galtier movie theater marquee suspended against the wall to your right. The movie theater has long been closed, but the marquee is kept brightly lit nonetheless.

● Enter the 375 Jackson skyway at the end of the building and go straight. This skyway offers a view of St. Paul's Lowertown outskirts. On your left you can see the former

First National Bank Building—the gigantic red "1" prominently displayed on top of the building makes a handy landmark for navigating downtown St. Paul.

- Go through the next skyway to enter the First National Bank/U.S. Bank Building. Take the second right to walk alongside the marble wall at the end of the walkway. Follow the path around to the 5th St. Center/Minnesota St. skyway entrance.

- Go through the skyway to the Alliance Bank Center. Take the left-hand path and go straight.

- Just before the escalators, turn right to enter the Town Square/6th St. skyway and go straight.

- Follow the path to your right and make a left at the dining court. Here you'll find La Loma Tamales, which makes its tamales from scratch, including grinding its own corn for the masa dough. Turn left again and walk toward Macy's (follow the overhead directional signs). Go straight into the Wells Fargo Place building.

- Turn right at the ATM and go to the left of the escalator and into the Wells Fargo atrium.

- Turn left to exit the building onto Wabasha St. N. Across the street is the Palace Theatre, the only vaudeville house in St. Paul that was not demolished. Charlie Chaplin, George Burns, and the Marx Brothers all appeared on the Palace's stage during its heyday, while the local comedy troupe, the Brave New Workshop, keeps the tradition of live theater alive today.

- Cross the street and turn right to follow Wabasha St. N. past neighborhood favorite Candyland, in this location since 1932. Don't miss the delicious warm gummy bears. Down the street you can see the back of the Fitzgerald Theater, St. Paul's oldest theater and the original home of the *Prairie Home Companion* radio show.

- Turn left at 7th St. W. to walk by the Minnesota Children's Museum. Go straight to the corner. Across the street from here, you'll see the distinctive Art Deco shape of Mickey's Diner, which has appeared in such movies as *Mighty Ducks I, II,* and *III;*

Jingle All the Way; and A *Prairie Home Companion.* Across the street is Church of the Assumption, built in 1874.

● Turn left on St. Peter St. and go straight. At 444 and 448 St. Peter St. are the former Coney Island Restaurant buildings—number 448 is the oldest building in St. Paul still located on its original site, constructed in 1858 as the state arsenal.

● Turn right at the Seventh Place Arch, going south to follow Washington St. past the impressive Romanesque-Châteauesque-style Landmark Center building. The Landmark Center was built in 1902 and originally served as the federal courthouse and a post office. Now a cultural center for the area, it was once the site of notable St. Paul gangster trials, including the one held for Alvin "Creepy" Karpis.

● Cross 5th St. W. and then cross Washington St. into Rice Park. Originally plotted in 1849 by the early developers of St. Paul, this park is the site of the first electric streetlights in St. Paul—installed to celebrate the completion of the Northern Pacific Railroad's line to the West Coast. Surrounding the park are some of the most impressive downtown St. Paul historic buildings, including the opulent St. Paul Hotel, the James J. Hill Reference and St. Paul Central Libraries, and the Ordway Center for the Performing Arts.

● After you've explored the park, continue to the corner of 5th St. W. and Market St., and turn left. Walk past Landmark Center and go straight across 6th St. W. Turn right into the Seventh Place Arch and go straight through the courtyard.

St. Paul Central Library

- Enter the Wells Fargo building at 430 Wabasha St. N. and go straight. Take the first left and make a right at the overlook.

- Turn left into the Town Square building and go straight.

- Turn right at the dining court and take the right path just before the escalator.

- Enter the skyway to Alliance Bank Center and follow the path to the left.

- Turn left at the escalators and go straight through to the skyway exit.

- Enter the U.S. Bank Building and take the path to your left. Follow the path to the U.S. Bank Center sign, and then take the left path to the 375 Jackson Building.

- Enter the skyway to the 375 Jackson Building. Go straight into the next skyway and then into Galtier Plaza.

- Go straight past the escalators and all the way to the big bank of windows on the other side of the building. Take the escalator down to the dining court.

- Turn right at the bottom of the escalator, go down the hall, and exit the building.

- Turn left to head toward the corner of 6th St. E. and Sibley St.

- Turn right and cross the street to Mears Park, our starting point. Across the street is Barrio Tequila Bar, an extraordinary Mexican restaurant with items such as soft-shell crab and mahimahi tacos.

POINTS OF INTEREST

Mears Park tinyurl.com/mearspark, 221 5th St. E., St. Paul, MN 55101, 651-632-5111

Galtier Plaza galtierplaza.com, 380 Jackson St., St. Paul, MN 55101

La Loma Tamales lalomatamales.com, 444 Cedar St., Ste. 210, St. Paul, MN 55101, 651-202-3153

Palace Theatre cinematreasures.org/theaters/2545, 17 7th Pl. W., St. Paul, MN 55102, 651-332-6620

Candyland candylandstore.com, 435 Wabasha St. N., St. Paul, MN 55102, 651-292-1191

Fitzgerald Theater fitzgeraldtheater.publicradio.org, 10 Exchange St. E., St. Paul, MN 55101, 651-290-1200

Minnesota Children's Museum mcm.org, 10 7th St. W., St. Paul, MN 55102, 651-225-6000

Mickey's Dining Car mickeysdiningcar.com, 36 7th St. W., St. Paul, MN 55102, 651-698-0259

Church of the Assumption assumptionsp.org, 51 7th St. W., St. Paul, MN 55102, 651-224-7536

Landmark Center landmarkcenter.org, 75 5th St. W., St. Paul, MN 55102, 651-292-3225

Rice Park tinyurl.com/ricepark, 109 4th St. W., St. Paul, MN 55102, 651-266-6400

James J. Hill Reference Library jjhill.org, 80 4th St. W., St. Paul, MN 55102, 651-265-5500

St. Paul Central Public Library tinyurl.com/stpaulcentrallibrary, 90 4th St. W., St. Paul, MN 55102, 651-266-7000

Ordway Center for the Performing Arts ordway.org, 345 Washington St., St. Paul, MN 55102, 651-282-3000

Barrio Tequila Bar barriotequila.com, 235 East 6th St., St. Paul, MN 55101, 651-222-3250

route summary

1. Start at the corner of 6th St. E. and Sibley St., and cross Sibley St. going southwest.
2. Turn left to get to the Galtier Plaza entrance on Sibley St. across from Mears Park.
3. Enter Galtier Plaza. Go straight, and then turn left just before the set of short stairs and take the escalator to the second floor.
4. Make a right to go around the top of the escalator and head straight down the hall.
5. Enter the 375 Jackson skyway at the end of the building and go straight.
6. Go through the next skyway to enter the First National Bank/U.S. Bank Building.
7. Take the second right at the marble wall at the end of the walkway.
8. Follow the path around to the 5th St. Center/Minnesota St. skyway entrance.
9. Go through the skyway to the Alliance Bank Center. Take the left-hand path and go straight.
10. Turn right before the escalators to enter the Town Square/6th St. skyway.

11. Enter the Town Square building and go straight.

12. Follow the path to your right and make a left at the dining court.

13. Turn left again and walk toward Macy's (see overhead directional signs). Go straight into the Wells Fargo Place building.

14. Turn right at the ATM, and go to the left of the escalator and into the Wells Fargo atrium.

15. Turn left to exit the building onto Wabasha St. N.

16. Cross the street and turn right to follow Wabasha St. N.

17. Turn left at 7th St. W. Go straight to the corner.

18. Turn left on St. Peter St. and go straight.

19. Turn right at the Seventh Place Arch and go straight to follow Washington St.

20. Cross 5th St. W. and Washington St. to enter Rice Park.

21. Go to the corner of 5th St. W. and Market St., and turn left. Walk past Landmark Center and go straight across 6th St. W.

22. Turn right into the Seventh Place Arch and go straight through the courtyard.

23. Enter the Wells Fargo building at 430 Wabasha St. N. and go straight. Take the first left and make a right at the overlook.

24. Turn left into the Town Square/Cedar Street Building and go straight.

25. Turn right at the dining court and take the right path just before the escalators.

26. Enter the skyway to Alliance Bank Center and follow the path to the left.

27. Turn left at the escalators and go straight through to the skyway exit.

28. Enter the U.S. Bank Building and take the path to your left. Follow the path to the U.S. Bank Center sign, and take the left path to the 375 Jackson Building.

29. Enter the skyway to the 375 Jackson Building. Go straight into the next skyway and then into Galtier Plaza.

30. Go straight past the escalators and all the way to the big bank of windows on the other side of the building. Take the escalator down to the dining court.

31. Turn right at the bottom of the escalator, go down the hall, and exit the building.

32. Turn left to head toward the corner of 6th St. E. and Sibley St.

33. Turn right and cross the street to Mears Park, our starting point.

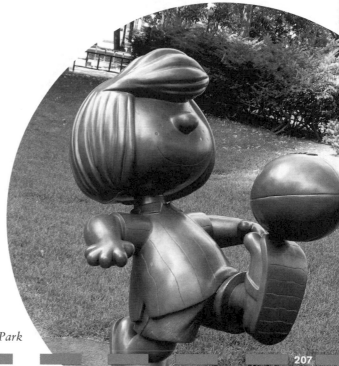

Peppermint Patty at Rice Park

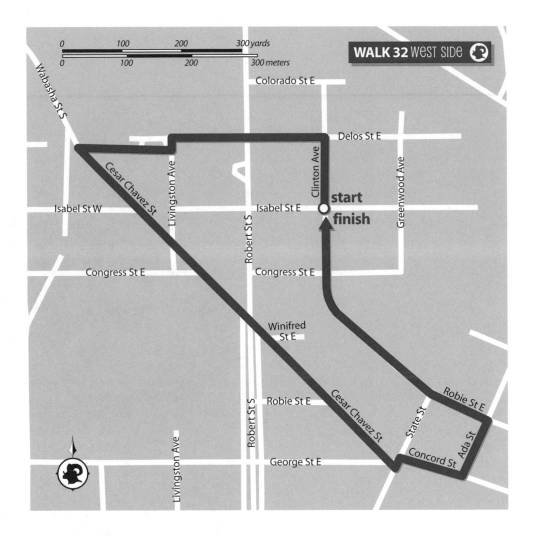

0   100   200   300 yards
0   100   200   300 meters

Colorado St E

Wabasha St S

Delos St E

Cesar Chavez St

Livingston Ave

Clinton Ave

Greenwood Ave

Isabel St W

Isabel St E

start
finish

Robert St S

Congress St E

Congress St E

Winifred
St E

Robert St S

Robie St E

Cesar Chavez St

Robie St E

State St

Ada St

Livingston Ave

George St E

Concord St

32 WEST SIDE: ETHNIC PAST MEETS ETHNIC RENAISSANCE

BOUNDARIES: Cesar Chavez St., Ada St., Clinton Ave., Robie St. E., Delos St. E.
HUDSON'S TWIN CITY STREET ATLAS COORDINATES: **Map 423, 2A**
DISTANCE: **Approx. 1 mile**
DIFFICULTY: **Easy**
PARKING: **Free parking on Congress St. and Clinton Ave.**
PUBLIC TRANSIT: **Bus lines 67, 68, and 75**

Directly south of downtown St. Paul and across the Mississippi River, the West Side is a geographic misnomer and an interesting historical and present-day neighborhood. It was settled after the first Wabasha Street Bridge was completed in 1859 but was not annexed by the city until 1874. The river was then a filthy industrial area prone to flooding, so, not surprisingly, the West Side was settled by a mix of poor ethnic groups. The Jewish community accounted for more than 70% of the neighborhood's population in 1915. Once significantly larger as the West Side Flats, the size of the business and residential area was reduced by urban renewal and later transformed into an industrial park.

In recent years, the area has transformed into St. Paul's largest Chicano business district, known as the District del Sol. St. Michael's Catholic Church, originally an Italian congregation, became the Torre de San Miguel Homes in 1968. A few years earlier, the Frias family opened Boca Chica, the still-thriving Mexican restaurant. More recently, Concord Ave. was renamed Cesar Chavez St. The area is multilayered with ethnic history, which continues through the bilingual businesses today. The neighborhood has played a pivotal role in St. Paul's history, and its prime location suggests that it will continue to do so.

● **Start on the corner of Isabel St. E. and Clinton Ave., and walk north on Clinton Ave. On the left are the gorgeous Isabel Apartments (109–119 Isabel St. E.). The row houses were constructed in 1904 beside an immense old cottonwood tree that stands behind the building.**

- Turn left on the pedestrian path and then continue west on Delos St. E. The bridge crosses Robert St. S. and provides a panoramic view of the St. Paul skyline to the north. After crossing the bridge, you'll come to the Torre de San Miguel Homes, a housing project from the late '60s that has undergone several renovations. It's home to a diverse group of immigrants from all over the world, most notably Mexico, Somalia, and Laos.

- Turn left on Livingston Ave. at the cul-de-sac, and then turn right immediately on Delos St. and continue west. On the right is the Torre de San Miguel, once the tower for St. Michael's Catholic Church, an Italian church built in 1882. The tower is the oldest remaining piece of architecture from the historic West Side Flats neighborhood.

- Continue forward, walking up the steps. On the right is the brick Colorado Street Bridge, built in 1888. It has served as a pedestrian-only bridge for a number of years.

- Turn left on Cesar Chavez St. This is the heart of the District del Sol. Boca Chica Restaurante Mexicano and Cantina has served an enormous menu of standard Mexican fare since 1964. The restaurant has grown over the years with the economic and cultural reemergence of the West Side.

- Cross Robert St. S., an intersection filled with Mexican American businesses and, toward the hill, a colorful sun mural. Ahead on the left is Parque de Castillo, a neighborhood park that hosts a summer music-and-movies series.

- Cross State St. to follow Cesar Chavez St. On the left is El Burrito Mercado, established in 1979. The Mexican American market, restaurant (El Café Restaurant), and deli predated the emergence of the West Side Chicano community. It offers reasonably priced, authentic Mexican food, such as tamales, tacos, chicken mole, homemade salsas, a wide selection of imported Mexican cheeses, fresh meats and seafood, and myriad other items. Across the street El Amanecer, a homey and inexpensive Mexican restaurant, offers a full menu of south-of-the-border favorites.

- Turn left on Ada St. On the right is the Holy Family Maronite Church, a Lebanese church, where a supper is occasionally served in this sea of Chicano culture. Historically, Lebanese often settled near Jewish populations, and today this is one of the few reminders of their presence here.

- Continue straight across Robie St. E. and turn left. On the right side is the Paul and Sheila Wellstone Center for Community building. The community center, completed in 2005, was named in honor of Minnesota's great liberal Democratic Senator Paul Wellstone and his wife, Sheila, who both died in a plane crash in 2002. Neighborhood House, its predecessor, was founded by Mount Zion Temple for immigrants in 1900.

- After passing the multilingual murals on the Wellstone Center, Robie St. E. merges into Clinton Ave. Continue north along the street to pass Parque de Castillo.

- Continue straight, heading north, and finish the walk at the intersection of Isabel St. E.

POINTS OF INTEREST

Boca Chica Restaurante Mexicano and Cantina
bocachicarestaurant.com, 11 Cesar Chavez St., St. Paul, MN 55107, 651-222-8499

Parque de Castillo tinyurl.com/parquedecastillo, 149 Cesar Chavez St., St. Paul, MN 55107, 651-632-5111

El Burrito Mercado elburritomercado.com, 175 Cesar Chavez St., St. Paul, MN 55107, 651-291-0758

El Amanecer 194 Cesar Chavez St., St. Paul, MN 55107, 651-291-0758

Holy Family Maronite Church holyfamilymaronitechurch.org, 203 Robie St. E., St. Paul, MN 55107, 651-291-1116

Torre de San Miguel

route summary

1. Start on the corner of Isabel St. E. and Clinton Ave. and walk north on Clinton Ave.
2. Turn left on the pedestrian path and then walk straight on Delos St. E.
3. Turn left on Livingston Ave. at the cul-de-sac, and turn immediately right on Delos St.
4. Continue west, walking up the steps.
5. Turn left on Cesar Chavez St.
6. Turn left on Ada St.
7. Cross Robie St. E. and turn left. After passing the Wellstone Center, Robie St. E. merges into Clinton Ave.
8. Continue straight to Isabel St. E. and finish the walk.

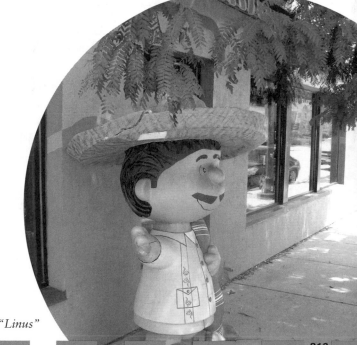

El Burrito Mercado's "Linus"

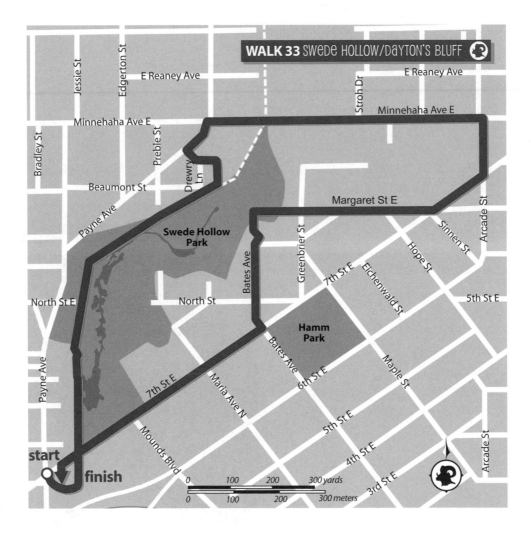

Jessie St

Edgerton St

E Reaney Ave

E Reaney Ave

Stroh Dr

Minnehaha Ave E

Bradley St

Minnehaha Ave E

Preble St

Drewry Ln

Beaumont St

Margaret St E

Arcade St

Payne Ave

Swede Hollow Park

Sinnen St

Greenbrier St

Hope St

7th St E

Eichenwald St

5th St E

North St E

North St

Bates Ave

Hamm Park

Maple St

Payne Ave

7th St E

Bates Ave

6th St E

5th St E

Arcade St

Maria Ave N

4th St E

start

Mounds Blvd

3rd St E

finish

0   100   200   300 yards

0   100   200   300 meters

33 SWEDE HOLLOW/DAYTON'S BLUFF: THE WORKING CLASS MOVES UP TO THE BLUFFS

BOUNDARIES: 6th St. E., Payne Ave., Minnehaha Ave. E., Arcade St.
HUDSON'S TWIN CITY STREET ATLAS **COORDINATES: Map 396, 2C and 2D**
DISTANCE: Approx. 2 miles
DIFFICULTY: Moderate
PARKING: Parking lots on Payne Ave. and 7th St. E.
PUBLIC TRANSIT: Bus line 74

Long before building codes and neighborhood zoning laws, Swedish immigrants first settled in what was then a marginal, flood-prone piece of land east of downtown St. Paul, in a small valley they called Svenska Dalen. For more than 100 years Swede Hollow, as it became known, was home to thousands of poor immigrant families living in essentially slum conditions—first Swedes, then Italians, and, in the last days of Swede Hollow, Mexicans—until the city condemned the area in the 1950s' throes of urban renewal.

While the hundreds of houses that once filled Swede Hollow are gone, you'll occasionally see a squared cluster of bricks that mark where a house once stood. All along the upper cliffs of the area stand the successful businesses started by the former residents of Swede Hollow—most notably James Morelli, whose descendants still own the wonderful Morelli's Italian deli and liquor store; and Gentille Yarusso, whose descendants own Yarusso-Bros. Italian Restaurant.

● **Enter the curlicue of the Bruce Vento Trailhead and follow the path down to the first fork, into Swede Hollow.**

● **Make a left at the bottom of the hill and follow the path under the set of picturesque stone bridges directly ahead—the 7th Street Improvement Arches. These bridges, built in 1884, are the only known examples of bridges constructed according to the helicoidal, or spiral method, in Minnesota; only a few other examples exist elsewhere in the United States.**

- Follow the path through the woods. On your right is Phalen Creek, which is home to many native species of birds, including ducks, egrets, herons, and Canada geese.

  At the first green bench, notice the steps leading down to the creek on your right. The valley below you is the former site of the Swede Hollow community. Scant evidence of it remains along the creek, but it's worth your while to go down the steps to investigate.

- Continue along the Bruce Vento Trail. At the first fork in the trail—look for the Payne Avenue Business District signpost on your right—turn left to go under the white bridge. This path will take you up to street level. This white tunnel is also significant because it's the only road in or out of Swede Hollow.

- Head up the hill and turn right at the SWEDE HOLLOW PARK sign. Follow the alley to Payne Ave.

- Go right on Payne Ave. and continue north.

- Turn right when you get to Minnehaha Ave. E. to walk past the amazing old Hamm's Brewery fortress at 690 Minnehaha Ave. E. If you're over 40 years old, you might remember seeing the Hamm's Bear beer commercials when you were a kid. The old commercials are now shown for camp effect in art theaters and at film festivals. On the right-hand corner of Minnehaha Ave. E. and Stroh Dr., notice the brick platform with spigots. This is the spot where Hamm's high-quality mineral water could be freely collected. Up until a decade ago, the spigots were still in use, and people would show up here with carloads of empty milk jugs to fill from the taps. About two blocks ahead is the site of the 1951 3M explosion, which killed 15 people and injured 50 more.

- Turn right on Arcade St. and go straight, heading south. If you like authentic Mexican food, this is a good place to take a break. Taqueria Los Paisanos has excellent Mexican fare, including reasonably priced seafood. Across the street, Mañana Restaurante y Pupuseria is the place to stop for Salvadoran food, including homemade empanadas and wonderful corn *pupusas,* the national dish of El Salvador.

eDWarD PHeLaN: NOTOrIOUS earLY seTTLer

Edward Phelan (whose name was variously spelled Phalen and Felyn) was a landowner who affixed his name to many pieces of property around his cabin, including Lake Phalen and Phalen Creek. Phelan was also the first person in St. Paul to be accused of murder, after his business partner, John Hays, was killed in 1839. Phelan himself was killed by his traveling companions in "self-defense" when he fled the state to evade prosecution. Local historian John Fletcher Williams wrote in 1876: "It is a disgrace, that the name of this brutal murderer has been affixed to one of our most beautiful lakes."

- Turn right on 7th St. E. and go straight southwest.

- Turn right at the Mexican Consulate building at the corner of Sinnen St. and 7th St. E., and go west down Margaret St. E. to Hamm Park. This park is the former site of Hamm Mansion, home of Theodore and Luisgarits Hamm, who started the Hamm Brewing Company in 1865.

- At the far left-hand corner of the park, you'll find a set of stairs. Take the stairs down to Bates Ave.

- Turn right to go straight on Bates Ave., past the STOP sign, and through the little neighborhood park at North St. E. and Bates Ave. At the left-hand side of the park is Swede Hollow Café, a great stop for a cup of coffee and a bite to eat.

- Turn right on 7th St. E. and go straight, heading southwest. Continue on until you reach Mounds Blvd.

- Cross the street and continue walking until you reach Payne Ave. Turn left into the parking lot to finish the walk.

POINTS OF INTEREST

Swede Hollow Park swedehollow.org or tinyurl.com/swedehollow, 615 7th St. E., St. Paul, MN 55106, 651-632-5111

Taqueria Los Paisanos 825 7th St. E., St. Paul, MN 55106, 651-778-8062

Mañana Restaurante y Pupuseria 828 7th St. E., St. Paul, MN 55106, 651-793-8482

Hamm Park tinyurl.com/hammpark, 743 7th St. E., St. Paul, MN 55106, 651-632-5111

Swede Hollow Café swedehollowcafe.com, 725 7th St. E., St. Paul, MN 55106, 651-776-8810

ROUTE SUMMARY

1. Enter the Bruce Vento Trail. Make a left at the bottom of the hill.

2. At the first fork in the trail, make a left to go under the white bridge.

3. Go uphill and turn right at the SWEDE HOLLOW PARK sign. Follow the alley to Payne Ave.

4. Go right on Payne Ave. and continue north.

5. Turn right when you get to Minnehaha Ave. E.

6. Turn right on Arcade St. and go south.

7. Turn right on 7th St. E. and go straight, heading southwest.

8. Turn right at the Mexican Consulate building (corner of Sinnen St. and 7th St. E.), and go west down Margaret St. E. to Swede Hollow Park.

9. At the left-hand corner of the park, take the stairs down to Maury St. and Bates Ave. Turn right to walk south down Bates Ave.

10. Turn right on 7th St. E. and go straight. Continue southwest until you reach Payne Ave., and turn left into the parking lot.

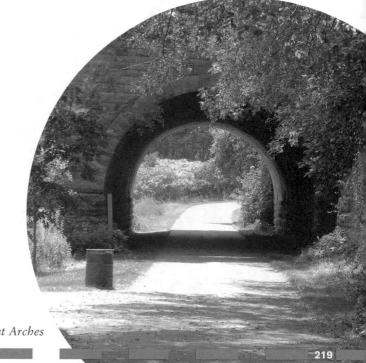

7th Street Improvement Arches

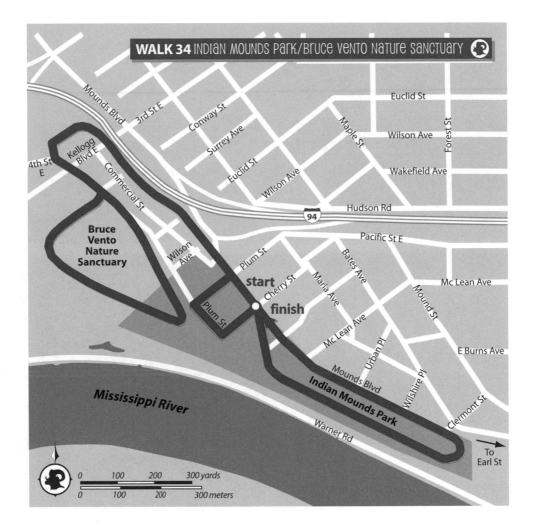

WALK 34 INDIAN MOUNDS PARK/BRUCE VENTO NATURE SANCTUARY

Euclid St

Wilson Ave

Forest St

Mounds Blvd

3rd St E

Conway St

Surrey Ave

Maple St

Euclid St

Wilson Ave

Wakefield Ave

4th St E

Kellogg Blvd E

Commercial St

94

Hudson Rd

Pacific St E

Bruce Vento Nature Sanctuary

Wilson Ave

Plum St

start

Cherry St

Bates Ave

Mc Lean Ave

Plum St

Maria Ave

finish

Mound St

Mc Lean Ave

Urban Pl

E Burns Ave

Mounds Blvd

Wilshire Pl

Indian Mounds Park

Clermont St

Mississippi River

Warner Rd

To Earl St

0   100   200   300 yards

0   100   200   300 meters

34 INDIAN MOUNDS Park/Bruce Vento Nature Sanctuary: Nature, Cityscapes, & History

BOUNDARIES: **Warner Rd., 4th St. E., Mounds Blvd., Clemont St.**
HUDSON'S TWIN CITY STREET ATLAS COORDINATES: **Map 396, 3D**
DISTANCE: **Approx. 4 miles**
DIFFICULTY: **Strenuous**
PARKING: **Free parking in the Indian Mounds Park parking lot, located at Cherry St. and Mounds Blvd.**
PUBLIC TRANSIT: **Bus line 74**

Established in 1893, Indian Mounds Park is one of the oldest parks in St. Paul. The park's name comes from the American Indian burial mounds that were found here by early settlers. These included 2,000-year-old Hopewell mounds, while others were constructed by the Dakota much later. Originally, there were 36 mounds in the park, but due to shortsighted construction projects and vandalism, only 6 remain in the park today.

At the far perimeter is the Bruce Vento Nature Sanctuary, the newest addition to the park. In the sanctuary, you'll be treated to sights of native birds and prairie grass, the previously inaccessible Carver's Cave and Brewer's Cave, as well as close-up views of freight trains rumbling down the same rails they've traversed for nearly 100 years. Pack a lunch for this walk—you won't find anywhere to buy food along this route, but you will find plenty of scenic places to stop and have a picnic.

● Begin at the Indian Mounds parking lot, located at Cherry St. and Mounds Blvd. Follow the sidewalk to your right, facing the overlook. From here, your vantage point gives you a scenic view of downtown St. Paul; the state capitol building; the Roberts, Wabasha, and High Bridges; the curve of the Mississippi River; and old railway beds.

● Turn left at the corner of Mounds. Blvd. and Plum St. onto the walking path. Follow the path downhill to parallel Commercial St.

- At the STOP sign at the bottom of the hill, cross the street at 4th St. E. and Commercial St. Follow the curve of the park entrance heading southeast. Go straight down 4th St. E. and make your first left into the Bruce Vento Nature Sanctuary parking lot.

- Go straight, heading southeast, through the short parking lot and onto the sanctuary trail. The sanctuary is home to many common and uncommon native birds, including bald eagles, northern flickers, great blue herons, and red-tailed hawks. Native species of flora are also planted here on these grounds, a project maintained by Minnesota's East Side Youth Conservation Corps. At the trailhead, informative markers provide the history of the area, as well as bird-identifying guides for bird-watchers.

- Go straight past the first fork in the path as it curves to the northeast. Occasionally, trains rumble past this area, and the trail offers lots of places to catch a closer look at them.

- Stay on the path closest to the bluffs as it moves southeast, and head up the bluffs to the oak woodland restoration area. Many lovely old trees—both dead and alive, and home to downy woodpeckers and other birds—are found along this part of the path. New trees have been planted here with the hopes that someday this will resemble, once again, the oak forest before the railways came through.

- Continue southeast. Just past the fork and on your left is Brewer's Cave, which, if you're a beer connoisseur, you might recognize from the picture on the Brewer's Cave Beer label. The pure stream coming from the rocks maintains a fairly constant temperature year-round—meaning this fount is one of the first places where you'll see green plants growing in the early days of spring. The little creek empties over a tiny, picturesque water-fall and into a nice-size pond—home to nesting waterbirds, including Canada geese, wood ducks, and mallards, and a hunting ground for kingfishers, herons, and egrets.

- Continue southeast on the path closest to the bluffs. On your left, you'll pass a great wall of exposed yellow sandstone and terra-cotta limestone blocks, as well as another large pond full of fish, birds, and muskrats. At the far end of the pond, you can see the walled-up remains of Wakan Tipi/Carver's Cave, which is the birthplace of the Dakota (more commonly known by the derogatory name the Sioux), according to their creation story. The front part of the cave was destroyed in the 1860s during railroad magnate James J. Hill's various construction projects, as were ancient petro-glyphs that filled the entrance of the cave. It was boarded up in the 1970s due to the Dakotas' wish to prevent further desecration of the cave.

● Turn around and take the path closest to the train tracks, headed northwest.

● Continue northwest all the way past the pond. All along the path are hundreds of native wildflowers and plants, including tiny daisylike dogbanes, yellow black-eyed Susans, and giant purple coneflowers.

● Go left past the second pond and the floodplain forest restoration area, headed southwest.

● Go straight past the next fork to walk up close to the train tracks. Some of the oldest and largest trees in the sanctuary are in this area. Follow the path as it curves to the right, northwest.

● At the next fork in the path, turn right. Turn left at the next fork and go straight.

● Exit the sanctuary and go straight through the parking lot. Turn right at the street and cross at the STOP sign. Turn left at the TO MOUNDS BLVD. sign and onto the walking path.

● Follow the path uphill. At the STOP sign at the top of the hill, cross the park exit at Cherry St. and make a right at the INDIAN MOUNDS PARK sign. Follow the path along the overlook and stay to the right to follow Mounds Blvd.

● Take a right at the next fork to walk alongside the scenic overlook. Below and to the right are more great views of St. Paul and the Mississippi River, as well as Holman Field, a small airstrip from which small private and military planes regularly take off. Down on the river, gigantic freight barges pass by with their loads, much as they've done since the 19th century.

● Stay to the right all the way up the hill and toward the beacon on its highest point.

● Just before you reach the beacon, take a right and an immediate left to continue up the steep hill. This takes you alongside the "airway" beacon for Holman Field. The beacon was built in 1929 to assist airmail delivery for the U.S. Postal Service planes leaving Holman Field.

- Go straight on the path to see the Indian Mounds, the park's namesake. Until the early 1980s, you could walk around on these mounds. To protect them from further damage, the iron gates were erected. These mounds were once much larger, but they were leveled during ill-conceived construction and landscaping projects in the late 19th century.

- Turn right at the second mound to follow the retaining wall. Follow the path past the third and fourth mounds, and then go straight to see the fifth and sixth mounds.

- After the sixth mound, turn left and continue around to your left. On your left is a big picnic pavilion, located at Mounds Blvd. and Earl St., which makes a great spot for eating your bag lunch.

- Go straight downhill on the combined bicycle/pedestrian path. In front of the beacon is a plaque about the structure, the last of its kind. On a clear day, you can see both downtown St. Paul and the Minneapolis skyline from here—look for the Minneapolis skyscrapers nestled between the Cathedral of Saint Paul and the state capitol.

- Go all the way down the hill until you get to the INDIAN MOUNDS sign at Cherry St. and Mounds Blvd.

- Turn left into the parking lot, and you're right back where you started.

POINT OF INTEREST:

Indian Mounds Park tinyurl.com/indianmoundsmn, 10 Mounds Blvd., St. Paul, MN 55106, 651-632-5111

Bruce Vento Nature Sanctuary nps.gov/miss/planyourvisit/ventosanctuary.htm, 4th St. E. and Commercial St., St. Paul, MN 55102, 651-266-6400

ROUTE SUMMARY

1. Begin at the Indian Mounds parking lot, located at Cherry St. and Mounds Blvd. Follow the sidewalk to your right, facing the overlook.

2. Turn left at the corner of Mounds. Blvd. and Plum St. onto the walking path. Follow the path downhill to parallel Commercial St.

3.   Cross the street at 4th St. E. and Commercial St. at the STOP sign at the bottom of the hill.

4.   Follow the curve of the park entrance to the left to go down 4th St. E. Make your first left into the Bruce Vento Nature Sanctuary parking lot.

5.   Go straight through the short parking lot and onto the sanctuary trail.

6.   Stay on the path closest to the bluffs, all the way past Brewer's Cave.

7.   At the end of the trail, at the pond in front of Wakan Tipi/Carver's Cave, turn around and take the path directly opposite of the one you came up on.

8.   Stay on the path closest to the train tracks, past the pond and the floodplain restoration area.

9.   Just after the floodplain restoration area, follow the path as it angles to the right.

10. Turn left at the next fork and go straight. Exit the sanctuary and go straight through the parking lot.

11. Turn right at the street and cross at the STOP sign. Turn left at the TO MOUNDS BLVD. sign and onto the walking path.

12. Follow the path up the hill. At the STOP sign at the top of the hill, cross the park exit at Cherry St. and make a right at the INDIAN MOUNDS PARK sign. Follow the path along the overlook and stay to the right to follow Mounds Blvd.

13. Take a right at the next fork to walk alongside the scenic overlook.

14. Stay to the right all the way up the hill and toward the beacon on its highest point.

15. Just before you reach the beacon, take a right and an immediate left to continue up the hill. Go straight on the path to see the Indian Mounds.

16. Turn right at the second mound to follow the retaining wall. Follow the path past the third and fourth mounds, and then go straight to see the fifth and sixth mounds.

17. After the sixth mound, turn left and continue around to your left.

18. Go straight down the hill on the combined bicycle/pedestrian path until you get to the INDIAN MOUNDS sign at Cherry St. and Mounds Blvd. to finish the walk.

Bruce Vento Nature Sanctuary

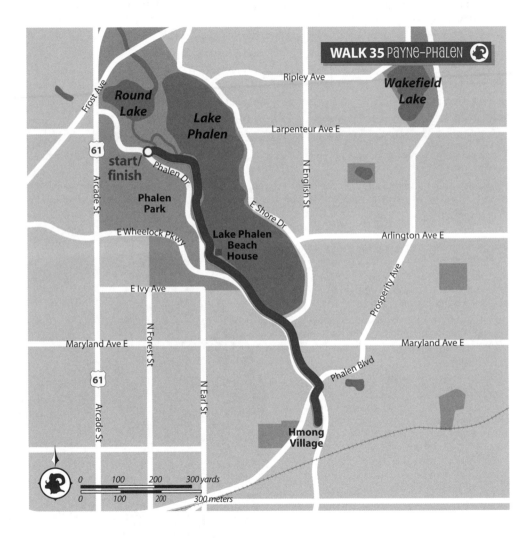

Ripley Ave

Wakefield Lake

Round Lake

Frost Ave

Lake Phalen

Larpenteur Ave E

61

start/finish

Phalen Dr

Phalen Park

N English St

E Shore Dr

Lake Phalen Beach House

E Wheelock Pkwy

Arlington Ave E

E Ivy Ave

N Forest St

Prosperity Ave

Maryland Ave E

61

Arcade St

N Earl St

Maryland Ave E

Phalen Blvd

Phalen Blvd

Hmong Village

0   100   200   300 yards

0   100   200   300 meters

35 Payne-Phalen: Picnic in the Park Southeast Asian-Style

BOUNDARIES: E. Ames Ave., Wheelock Pkwy., Phalen Dr., Frost Ave., East Shore Dr.
HUDSON'S TWIN CITY STREET ATLAS **COORDINATES: Map 396, 3B and 4B**
DISTANCE: Approx. 3¾ miles
DIFFICULTY: Moderate
PARKING: Free parking lot at the beginning of the walk
PUBLIC TRANSIT: Bus line 64

Over the years the ethnic dynamic of Payne–Phalen has changed—but the lake remains at its center. Located at the northern corner of the neighborhood and St. Paul (a portion extends into suburban Maplewood), Lake Phalen, the city's original water supply, was acquired in 1899. The 278-acre public park opened in time for the first wave of predominantly Swedish immigration, and each successive generation has swum at the swimming beach and picnicked in the park. The eastside neighborhood has remained solidly blue collar as Italians, Latinos, and, most recently, Mexicans and the Hmong from Southeast Asia arrived. The ethnic minority from Laos fought against the communist Pathet Lao during the Vietnam War. In 1975 the federal government recognized their service, and over four decades 250,000 Hmong moved to the U.S. Today only Minnesota trails California in total number of Hmong residents.

The annual Dragon Festival in July celebrates the area's wealth of pan-Asian culture. The two-day event includes food, music, arts, martial arts—and the dragon boat race. Based on competition originating in China more than 2,400 years ago, teams of 20 compete in colorful 40-by-4-foot boats rowing to a drumbeat as thousands of multigenerational spectators relax on the shores of Lake Phalen.

● Start at the northwesternmost parking lot and follow the innermost walking path down the hill and over the bridge.

● Cross the bridge over the creek connecting Round Lake and Lake Phalen. On your left is the statue *Meditation* by world-famous sculptor Lei Yixin of Changsu, China, a St. Paul sister city. Over the years he has created hundreds of public sculptures, ranging from Mao Zedong in China to the Martin Luther King Jr. National Memorial in Washington, D.C.

- Go under the bridge, keep to the left, and merge with bike path passing the playground and picnic pavilion.

- Follow the path immediately right after passing the memorial statue of the Civilian Conservation Corps, and stay in the pedestrian lane ascending the hill.

- Continue on the wending path passing Phalen Park Golf Course on the right across the street.

- Follow the pedestrian path around the Lake Phalen Beach House.

- Then continue on the walking path closest to the lake at the beach house—the only lakeside public-swimming beach in St. Paul.

- The path again merges with the bike lane, passing the watershed district's abundance of cattails and bird nests as it curves around the lake.

- Turn right, following the pedestrian path and walking away from the lake to the intersection of East Shore Dr. and Wheelock Pkwy./Johnson Pkwy. Then cross East Shore on Johnson Pkwy. Originally platted in Suburban Hills near the Mounds Park neighborhood, the street, it is speculated, was named in honor of surveyor Gates Johnson. In 1930 the street was extended into a parkway terminating at Lake Phalen and was rededicated in honor of John A. Johnson, who served as Minnesota governor 1905–1909. Of Swedish descent, he was the first Minnesota-born governor. At the 1908 Democratic Convention, he was nominated for president but lost to William Jennings Bryan. Tragically, he was the state's first governor to die in office.

- After crossing Phalen Blvd., on the left is Phalen Crossing, the heart of the city's Phalen Corridor revitalization, completed in 2004: 300 units of condos and townhomes stretched over 14 acres; a restored pond and roads replaced the site of a dilapidated eastside shopping mall.

- Turn right, crossing Johnson Pkwy., and turn left immediately, following the sidewalk.

- Continue a quarter mile. On the right is Hmong Village, a triumph of the American immigrant mom-and-pop business. The nondescript exterior of the former warehouse building belies what's inside: more than 230 merchant stalls with traditional Hmong clothing, CDs, DVDs, jewelry, groceries, a farmers market, and, of course, food—delicious food that will stuff a family of four for less than $25. The flavors of Southeast Asia: *pho, chow fun,* egg rolls, spring rolls, Hmong sausage, papaya salad, and so much more provide a yummy escape, regardless of the weather outside.

- When your visit to Hmong Village is over, turn around, turning left on Johnson Pkwy., and follow the path back to Phalen Blvd. Then turn right and then left on Johnson Pkwy.

- Cross East Shore Dr. and turn left, following the lake to the beach house.

- Follow the path right, crossing the parking lot along the lake.

- Descending the hill, follow the middle path passing the playground again and native wildflowers on the right as the path veers under the bridge.

- After crossing the bridge on the left across the creek and up the hill is the Ice Palace Plaque. The plaque commemorates the centennial of the St. Paul Winter Carnival in 1986; the ice structure included towers as high as 128 feet, and for the short time before it melted, it attracted more than a million visitors.

- Cross the next bridge and walk to the parking lot, our starting point.

POINTS OF INTEREST

Phalen Park tinyurl.com/phalenpark, 1600 Phalen Dr., St. Paul, MN 55106, 651-632-5111

Phalen Park Golf Course golfstpaul.org, 1615 Phalen Dr., St. Paul, MN 55106, 651-778-0413

Hmong Village 1001 Johnson Pkwy., St. Paul, MN 55106, 651-777-7886

ROUTE SUMMARY

1. Start at the northwesternmost parking lot, and follow the innermost walking path down the hill and over the bridge.

2. Cross the bridge over the creek.

3. Go under the bridge and keep to the left, merging with bike path passing the playground and picnic pavilion.

4. Follow the path immediately right after passing the memorial statue of the Civilian Conservation Corps, and stay in the pedestrian lane ascending the hill.

5. Continue on the wending path passing Phalen Park Golf Course.

6. Follow the pedestrian path around the Lake Phalen Beach House.

7. Then continue on the walking path closest to the lake at the beach house.

8. The path again merges with the bike lane, passing the watershed district as it curves around the lake.

9. Turn right, following the pedestrian path and walking away from the lake to the intersection of East Shore Dr. and Wheelock Pkwy./Johnson Pkwy. Then cross East Shore on Johnson Pkwy.

10. Turn right, crossing Johnson Pkwy., and turn left immediately, following the sidewalk.

11. Continue a quarter mile; on the right is Hmong Village.

12. When your visit is over at Hmong Village, turn around, turning left on Johnson Pkwy. Then follow the path back to Phalen Blvd., and turn right and then left on Johnson Pkwy.

13. Cross East Shore Dr. and turn left, following the lake to the beach house.

14. Follow the path right, crossing the parking lot along the lake.

15. Descending the hill, follow the middle path, passing the playground again as the path veers under the bridge.

16. Cross the first bridge.

17. Cross the second bridge, and walk to the parking lot, our starting point.

Lake Phalen

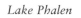

Appendix 1: WALKS BY THEME

NATURAL SPACES

Lake Calhoun (Walk 2)
Lake Harriet (Walk 3)
Loring Park & the Walker Art Center (Walk 7)
Bridge Square, the Gateway, Boom Island, Nicollet Island, & the North Loop (Walk 14)
Minnehaha Parkway/48th & Chicago (Walk 22)
Minnehaha Falls (Walk 23)
Highland Park & Hidden Falls Park (Walk 24)
Como Park (Walk 29)
Swede Hollow/Dayton's Bluff (Walk 33)
Indian Mounds Park/Bruce Vento Nature Sanctuary (Walk 34)
Payne-Phalen (Walk 35)

HISTORIC AREAS

Phillips & Elliot Park (Walk 6)
Minneapolis Downtown & Theatre District (Walk 10)
Nicollet Mall (Walk 11)
Downtown/Washington Avenue (Walk 12)
Warehouse District/North Loop (Walk 13)
Bridge Square, the Gateway, Boom Island, Nicollet Island, & the North Loop (Walk 14)
Historic Mill District (Walk 15)
East Hennepin/Marcy-Holmes (Walk 16)
U of M (Walk 18)
Nordeast Minneapolis (Walk 19)
Prospect Park's Tower Hill Park & Water Tower (Walk 20)
Minneapolis's Lake Street (Walk 21)
Minnehaha Falls (Walk 23)
Cathedral, Ramsey, & Summit Hills (Walk 26)
Crocus Hill (Walk 27)
Minnesota State Capitol (Walk 28)
Downtown St. Paul (Walk 31)
Swede Hollow/Dayton's Bluff (Walk 33)
Indian Mounds Park/Bruce Vento Nature Sanctuary (Walk 34)

DINING, SHOPPING, AND ENTERTAINMENT

Uptown (Walk 1)
Nicollet Avenue's Eat Street (Walk 4)
Cedar-Riverside (Walk 8)
Downtown Minneapolis (Walk 9)
Minneapolis Downtown & Theatre District (Walk 10)

Nicollet Mall (Walk 11)
Downtown/Washington Avenue (Walk 12)
East Hennepin/Marcy-Holmes (Walk 16)
Dinkytown (Walk 17)
Nordeast Minneapolis (Walk 19)
Minneapolis's Lake Street (Walk 21)
Minnehaha Parkway/48th & Chicago
(Walk 22)
Highland Park & Hidden Falls Park
(Walk 24)
Grand Avenue (Walk 25)
Cathedral, Ramsey, & Summit Hills
(Walk 26)
Irvine Park & West 7th Street (Walk 30)
Downtown St. Paul (Walk 31)
West Side (Walk 32)
Swede Hollow/Dayton's Bluff (Walk 33)
Payne-Phalen (Walk 35)

around campus

Dinkytown (Walk 17)
U of M (Walk 18)
Grand Avenue (Walk 25)

architecture

Whittier (Walk 5)
Phillips & Elliot Park (Walk 6)
Loring Park & the Walker Art Center
(Walk 7)
Downtown Minneapolis (Walk 9)
Minneapolis Downtown & Theatre District
(Walk 10)
Nicollet Mall (Walk 11)
Downtown/Washington Avenue (Walk 12)
Warehouse District/North Loop (Walk 13)
Historic Mill District (Walk 15)
U of M (Walk 18)
Nordeast Minneapolis (Walk 19)
Crocus Hill (Walk 27)
Minnesota State Capitol (Walk 28)
Como Park (Walk 29)
Irvine Park & West 7th Street (Walk 30)
Downtown St. Paul (Walk 31)

Appendix 2: POINTS OF INTEREST

FOOD & DRINK

Acadia Café acadiacafe.com, 329 Cedar Ave. S., Minneapolis, 612-874-8702 (Walk 8)

Al's Breakfast 413 14th Ave. S.E., Minneapolis, 612-331-9991 (Walk 17)

Amy's Classic Confections skywaymyway.com, 601 Marquette Ave., Northstar Center, Minneapolis, 612-436-0016 (Walk 9)

Annie's Parlour facebook.com/dinkytownnannies, 313 14th Ave. S.E., Minneapolis, 612-379-0744 (Walk 17)

Aster Café aster-cafe.com, 121 Main St., Minneapolis, 612-379-3138 (Walk 15)

The Bachelor Farmer thebachelorfarmer.com, 50 North 2nd Ave., Minneapolis, 612-206-3920 (Walk 14)

Band Box Diner facebook.com/bandboxeats, 729 10th St. S., Minneapolis, 612-332-0850 (Walk 6)

Barbette barbette.com, 1600 Lake St. W., Minneapolis, 612-827-5710 (Walk 1)

Barrio Tequila Bar barriotequila.com, 235 East 6th St., St. Paul, 651-222-3250 (Walk 31)

Be'Wiched Deli bewicheddeli.com, 800 Washington Ave. N., Minneapolis, 612-767-4330 (Walk 13)

Black Forest Inn blackforestinnmpls.com, 1 26th St. E., Minneapolis, 612-872-0812 (Walk 4)

Black Sheep blacksheeppizza.com, 600 Washington Ave. N., Minneapolis, 612-342-2625 (Walk 13)

Boca Chica Restaurante Mexicano and Cantina bocachicarestaurant.com, 11 Cesar Chavez St., St. Paul, 651-222-8499 (Walk 32)

Brasa Rotisserie brasa.us, 600 Hennepin Ave. E., Minneapolis, 612-379-3030 (Walk 16)

Bravo! Café & Bakery bravobakery.net, 1106 Grand Ave., St. Paul, 651-287-9118 (Walk 25)

Brit's Pub britspub.com, 1110 Nicollet Mall, Minneapolis, 612-332-3908 (Walk 11)

Broder's Cucina Italiana broders.com, 2308 50th St. W., Minneapolis, 612-925-3113 (Walk 3)

Broder's Pasta broders.com, 5000 Penn Ave. S., Minneapolis, 612-925-9202 (Walk 3)

The Bulldog N.E. thebulldognortheast.com, 401 Hennepin Ave. E., Minneapolis, 612-378-2855 (Walk 16)

Café Latte cafelatte.com, 850 Grand Ave., St. Paul, 651-224-5687 (Walk 25)

Café Levain cafelevain.com, 4762 Chicago Ave. S., Minneapolis, 612-823-7111 (Walk 22)

Café Lurcat cafelurcat.com, 624 Harmon Pl., Minneapolis, 612-486-5500 (Walk 7)

Camdi Restaurant camdirestaurant.com, 1325 4th St. S.E., Minneapolis, 612-331-4194 (Walk 17)

Chatterbox Pub chatterboxpub.net, 800 Cleveland Ave., St. Paul, 651-699-1149 (Walk 24)

Cheng Heng Restaurant 448 University Ave. W., St. Paul, 651-222-5577 (Walk 28)

Chilly Billy's chillybillysfrozenyogurt.com, 314 15th Ave. SE, Minneapolis, 612-843-4278 (Walk 18)

Classic Cookie mplsclassiccookie.mysite.com, 200 5th St. S., #295, Wells Fargo Midland Building, Minneapolis, 612-338-1949 (Walk 9)

Cleveland Wok clevelandwok.com, 767 Cleveland Ave., St. Paul, 651-699-3141 (Walk 24)

Como Lakeside Pavilion tinyurl.com/comopavilion, 1360 Lexington Pkwy. N., St. Paul, 651-488-4920 (Walk 29)

Corner Coffee yourcornercoffee.com, 514 3rd St. N., #102, Minneapolis, 612-338-2002 (Walk 13)

Cossetta's Italian Market and Pizzeria/Louis Ristorante & Bar cossettas.com, 211 7th St. W., St. Paul, 651-222-3476 (Walk 30)

Cow Bella Gelato cowbellagelato.com, 1700 Grand Ave., St. Paul, 651-340-0585 (Walk 25)

Dakota Restaurant & Jazz Club dakotacooks.com, 1010 Nicollet Ave., Minneapolis, 612-332-1010 (Walk 11)

88 Oriental Foods 291 University Ave. W., St. Paul, 651-209-8388 (Walk 28)

El Amanecer 194 Cesar Chavez St., St. Paul, 651-291-0758 (Walk 32)

El Burrito Mercado elburritomercado.com, 175 Cesar Chavez St., St. Paul, 651-291-0758 (Walk 32)

Forepaugh's Restaurant forepaughs.com, 276 Exchange St. S., St. Paul, 651-224-5606 (Walk 30)

Freight House/Dunn Bros. Coffee freighthouse.dunnbros.com, 201 3rd Ave. S., Minneapolis, 612-692-8530 (Walk 12)

Fulton Brewery Tap Room fultonbeer.com, 414 6th Ave. N., Minneapolis, 612-333-3208 (Walk 13)

Gardens of Salonica gardensofsalonica.com, 19 5th St. N.E., Minneapolis, 612-378-0611 (Walk 16)

Gather gatherbydamico.com, 1750 Hennepin Ave., Minneapolis, 612-253-3400 (Walk 7)

Gluek's Restaurant & Bar glueks.com, 16 6th St. N., Minneapolis, 612-338-6621 (Walk 10)

Grandview Grill newgrandviewgrill.com, 1818 Grand Ave., St. Paul, 651-698-2346 (Walk 25)

Guayaquil 1526 Lake St. E., Minneapolis, 612-722-2346 (Walk 21)

Happy Gnome thehappygnome.com, 498 Selby Ave., St. Paul, 651-287-2018 (Walk 26)

Hard Times Café hardtimes.com, 1821 Riverside Ave., Minneapolis, 612-341-9261 (Walk 8)

Highland Café & Bakery highlandcafeonline.com, 2012 Ford Pkwy., St. Paul, 651-698-3400 (Walk 24)

Highland Grill highlandgrill.com, 771 Cleveland Ave., St. Paul, 651-690-1173 (Walk 24)

Hmong Village 1001 Johnson Pkwy., St. Paul, 651-777-7886 (Walk 35)

Jax Café jaxcafe.com, 1928 University Ave. N.E., Minneapolis, 612-789-7297 (Walk 19)

Jerusalem's Restaurant 1518 Nicollet Ave., Minneapolis, 612-871-8883 (Walk 4)

Joe's Garage joes-garage.com, 1610 Harmon Pl., Minneapolis, 612-904-1163 (Walk 7)

Kafe 421 kafe421.com, 421 14th Ave. S.E., Minneapolis, 612-623-4900 (Walk 17)

Kitty Cat Klub kittycatklub.net, 315 14th Ave. S.E., Minneapolis, 612-331-9800 (Walk 17)

Kramarczuk's kramarczuk.com, 215 Hennepin Ave. E., Minneapolis, 612-379-3018 (Walk 16)

La Belle Vie labellevie.us, 510 Groveland Ave., Minneapolis, 612-874-6440 (Walk 7)

La Loma Tamales lalomatamales.com, 444 Cedar St., Ste. 210, St. Paul, 651-202 3153 (Walk 31)

The Liffey Irish Pub theliffey.com, 175 7th St. W., St. Paul, 651-556-1420 (Walk 30)

Little Szechuan littleszechuan.com, 422 University Ave. W., St. Paul, 651-222-1333 (Walk 28)

Local Irish Pub the-local.com, 931 Nicollet Mall, Minneapolis, 612-904-1000 (Walk 11)

Loring Pasta Bar loringcafe.com, 327 14th Ave. S.E., Minneapolis, 612-378-4849 (Walk 17)

Mañana Restaurante y Pupuseria 828 7th St. E., St. Paul, 651-793-8482 (Walk 33)

Market Bar-B-Que marketbbq.com, 1414 Nicollet Ave., Minneapolis, 612-872-1111 (Walk 4)

Masa masa-restaurant.com, 1070 Nicollet Mall, Minneapolis, 612-338-6272 (Walk 11)

Mercado Central mercadocentral.net, 1515 Lake St. E., Minneapolis, 612-728-5401 (Walk 21)

Mesa Pizza Uptown mesapizzamn.com, 1440 Lake St. W., Minneapolis, 612-206-3206 (Walk 1)

Mickey's Dining Car mickeysdiningcar.com, 36 7th St. W., St. Paul, 651-698-0259 (Walk 31)

Midtown Global Market midtownglobalmarket.org, 2929 Chicago Ave. S., Minneapolis, 612-872-4041 (Walk 21)

Moscow on the Hill moscowonthehill.com, 371 Selby Ave., St. Paul, 651-291-1236 (Walk 26)

Muddy Pig muddypig.com, 162 Dale St., St. Paul, 651-254-1030 (Walk 26)

Nicollet Island Inn nicolletislandinn.com, 95 Merriam St., Minneapolis, 612-331-1800 (Walk 15)

Ngon Bistro ngonbistro.com, 799 University Ave. W., St. Paul, 651-222-3301 (Walk 28)

Nye's Polonaise Room nyespolonaise.com, 112 Hennepin Ave. E., Minneapolis, 612-379-2021 (Walk 16)

Origami Restaurant origamirestaurant.com, 30 1st St. N., Minneapolis, 612-333-8430 (Walk 14)

Pagoda pagodadinkytown.com, 1417 4th St. S.E., Minneapolis, 612-378-4710 (Walk 17)

Pancho Villa panchovillasgrill.com, 2539 Nicollet Ave., Minneapolis, 612-871-7014 (Walk 4)

Peninsula Malaysian Cuisine peninsulamalaysiancuisine.com, 2608 Nicollet Ave., Minneapolis, 612-871-8282 (Walk 4)

Pepito's Mexican Restaurant pepitosrestaurant.com, 4820 Chicago Ave. S., Minneapolis, 612-822-2104 (Walk 22)

Pho Tau Bay photaubay.us, 2837 Nicollet Ave., Minneapolis, 612-874-6030 (Walk 4)

Pizza Lucé pizzaluce.com, 119 4th St. N., Minneapolis, 612-333-7359 (Walk 13)

Pracna pracna.com, 117 Main St., Minneapolis, 612-379-3200 (Walk 15)

Pumphouse Creamery pumphouse-creamery.com, 4754 Chicago Ave. S., Minneapolis, 612-825-2021 (Walk 22)

Punch Neopolitan Pizza punchpizza.com, 210 Hennepin Ave. E., Minneapolis, 612-623-8114 (Walk 16)

Purple Onion Café thepurpleonioncafe.com, 1301 University Ave. S.E., Minneapolis, 612-252-0217 (Walk 17)

Quang quangrestaurant.com, 2719 Nicollet Ave., Minneapolis, 612-874-6030 (Walk 4)

Que Nha 849 University Ave. W., St. Paul, 651-290-8552 (Walk 28)

Rainbow Chinese Restaurant and Bar rainbowrestaurant.com, 2739 Nicollet Ave., Minneapolis, 612-870-7081 (Walk 4)

The Sample Room the-sample-room.com, 2124 Marshall St., Minneapolis, 612-789-0333 (Walk 19)

Sea Salt Eatery seasalteatery.wordpress.com, 4825 Minnehaha Ave., Minneapolis, 612-721-8990 (Walk 23)

Shish Mediterranean Grill and Café shishcafe.net, 1668 Grand Ave., St. Paul, 651-690-2212 (Walk 25)

Smack Shack smack-shack.com, 603 Washington Avenue N., Minneapolis, 612-379-4322 (Walk 13)

Spoonriver Restaurant spoonriver.com, 750 2nd St. S., Minneapolis, 612-436-2236 (Walk 15)

Spyhouse Espresso Bar and Gallery spyhousecoffeeshop.com, 2451 Nicollet Ave., Minneapolis, 612-871-3177 (Walk 4)

Stella's Fish Café & Prestige Oyster Bar stellasfishcafe.com, 1400 Lake St. W., Minneapolis, 612-824-8862 (Walk 1)

Stub and Herb's Bar and Restaurant stubandherbsbar.com, 227 Oak St. S.E., Minneapolis, 612-379-1880 (Walk 18)

Swede Hollow Café swedehollowcafe.com, 725 7th St. E., St. Paul, 651-776-8810 (Walk 33)

Taqueria La Hacienda taquerialahacienda.com, 1515 Lake St. E., #104, Minneapolis, 612-822-2715 (Walk 21)

Taqueria Los Paisanos 825 7th St. E., St. Paul, 651-778-8062 (Walk 33)

Tavern on Grand tavernongrand.com, 656 Grand Ave., St. Paul, 651-228-9030 (Walk 25)

Tea House ourteahouse.com, 330 2nd Ave. S., Towle Building, Minneapolis, 612-343-2133 (Walk 9)

TeaSource teasource.com, 752 Cleveland Ave., St. Paul, 651-690-9822 (Walk 24)

The Tin Fish thetinfish.net, 3000 Calhoun Pkwy. E., Minneapolis, 612-823-5840 (Walk 2)

Town Hall Tap townhallbrewery.com, 4810 Chicago Ave. S., Minneapolis, 612-767-7307 (Walk 22)

Triple Rock Social Club triplerocksocialclub.com, 629 Cedar Ave. S., Minneapolis, 612-333-7399 (Walk 8)

Tuggs Tavern tuggstavern.com, 219 Main St., Minneapolis, 612-379-4404 (Walk 15)

Tum Rup Thai tumrupthai.com, 1221 Lake St. W., Minneapolis, 612-824-1378 (Walk 1)

Turtle Bread Company turtlebread.com, 4782 Chicago Ave. S., Minneapolis, 612-823-7333 (Walk 22)

The Varsity Theater & Café des Artistes varsitytheater.org/cafe, 1308 4th St. S.E., Minneapolis, 612-604-0222 (Walk 17)

Vincent A Restaurant vincentarestaurant.com, 1100 Nicollet Mall, Minneapolis, 612-630-1189 (Walk 11)

W. A. Frost & Company wafrost.com, 374 Selby Ave., St. Paul, 651-324-5715 (Walk 26)

Wally's wallysfalafelandhummus.com, 423 14th Ave. S.E., Minneapolis, 612-746-4776 (Walk 17)

The Wienery wienery.com, 414 Cedar Ave. S., Minneapolis, 612-333-5798 (Walk 8)

Wilde Roast Cafe wilderoastcafe.com, 65 Main St. S.E., Minneapolis, 612-331-4544 (Walk 15)

Williams Uptown Pub & Peanut Bar williamsminneapolis.com, 2911 Hennepin Ave., Minneapolis, 612-823-6271 (Walk 1)

Zelo zelomn.com, 831 Nicollet Mall, Minneapolis, 612-333-7000 (Walk 11)

ENTERTAINMENT & NIGHTLIFE

Acadia Café acadiacafe.com, 329 Cedar Ave. S., Minneapolis, 612-874-8702 (Walk 8)

Brave New Workshop theatre.bravenewworkshop.com, 824 Hennepin Ave., Minneapolis, 612-332-6620 (Walk 10)

Brit's Pub britspub.com, 1110 Nicollet Mall, Minneapolis, 612-332-3908 (Walk 11)

Cedar Cultural Center thecedar.org, 416 Cedar Ave. S., Minneapolis, 612-338-2674 (Walk 8)

Chatterbox Pub chatterboxpub.net, 800 Cleveland Ave., St. Paul, 651-699-1149 (Walk 24)

Dakota Restaurant & Jazz Club dakotacooks.com, 1010 Nicollet Ave., Minneapolis, 612-332-1010 (Walk 11)

First Avenue and 7th Street Entry/The Depot Tavern first-avenue.com, 701 1st Ave. N., Minneapolis, 612-332-1775 (Walk 10)

Fitzgerald Theater fitzgeraldtheater.publicradio.org, 10 Exchange St. E., St. Paul, 651-290-1200 (Walk 31)

Gasthof zur Gemütlichkeit/Mario's Keller Bar gasthofzg.com, 2300 University Ave. N.E., Minneapolis, 612-781-3860 (Walk 19)

The Gay 90's gay90s.com, 408 Hennepin Ave., Minneapolis, 612-333-7755 (Walk 10)

Gluek's Restaurant & Bar glueks.com, 16 6th St. N., Minneapolis, 612-338-6621 (Walk 10)

Grumpy's grumpys-bar.com/downtown, 1111 Washington Ave. S., Minneapolis, 612-340-9738 (Walk 12)

Happy Gnome thehappygnome.com, 498 Selby Ave., St. Paul, 651-287-2018 (Walk 26)

Highland 2 Theatres manntheatresmn.com, 760 Cleveland Ave., St. Paul, 651-698-3085 (Walk 24)

Hubert H. Humphrey Metrodome msfc.com, 900 5th Ave. S., Minneapolis, 612-332-0386 (Walk 12)

Icehouse Restaurant icehousempls.com, 2528 Nicollet Ave., Minneapolis, 612-276-6523 (Walk 4)

In the Heart of the Beast Puppet and Mask Theatre hobt.org, 1500 Lake St. E., Minneapolis, 612-721-2535 (Walk 21)

Kitty Cat Klub kittycatklub.net, 315 14th Ave. S.E., Minneapolis, 612-331-9800 (Walk 17)

Lagoon Cinema landmarktheatres.com/market/minneapolis/lagooncinema.htm, 1320 Lagoon Ave., Minneapolis, 612-825-6006 (Walk 1)

Lake Harriet Bandshell tinyurl.com/harrietlake, 43rd St. W. and E. Lake Harriet Pkwy., Minneapolis (Walk 3)

The Liffey Irish Pub theliffey.com, 175 7th St. W., St. Paul, 651-556-1420 (Walk 30)

Local Irish Pub the-local.com, 931 Nicollet Mall, Minneapolis, 612-904-1000 (Walk 11)

Lure Showclub lurempls.com/the-club, 723 Hennepin Ave., Minneapolis, 612-333-2323 (Walk 10)

Mixed Blood Theatre mixedblood.com, 1501 4th St. S., Minneapolis, 612-338-0937 (Walk 8)

Muddy Pig muddypig.com, 162 Dale St., St. Paul, 651-254-1030 (Walk 26)

Nye's Polonaise Room nyespolonaise.com, 112 Hennepin Ave. E., Minneapolis, 612-379-2021 (Walk 16)

Orchestra Hall minnesotaorchestra.org, 1111 Nicollet Ave., Minneapolis, 612-371-5600 (Walk 11)

Ordway Center for the Performing Arts ordway.org, 345 Washington St., St. Paul, 651-282-3000 (Walk 31)

Orpheum Theatre hennepintheatretrust.org/our-theatres/orpheum-theatre, 910 Hennepin Ave., Minneapolis, 612-339-7007 (Walk 10)

Palace Theatre cinematreasures.org/theaters/2545, 17 7th Pl. W., St. Paul, 651-332-6620 (Walk 31)

Pantages Theatre hennepintheatretrust.org/our-theatres/pantages-theatre, 710 Hennepin Ave., Minneapolis, 612-373-5600 (Walk 10)

Pepito's Parkway Theater theparkwaytheater.com, 4814 Chicago Ave. S., Minneapolis, 612-822-3030 (Walk 22)

Patrick McGovern's Pub and Restaurant patmcgoverns.com, 225 7th St. W., St. Paul, 651-224-5821 (Walk 30)

Pracna pracna.com, 117 Main St., Minneapolis, 612-379-3200 (Walk 15)

Psycho Suzi's psychosuzis.com, 1900 Marshall Ave. N.E., Minneapolis, 612-788-9069 (Walk 19)

Red Stag Supperclub redstagsupperclub.com, 509 6th St. N.E., Minneapolis, 612-767-7766 (Walk 16)

Ritz Theater ritzdolls.com, 345 13th Ave. N.E., Minneapolis, 612-623-7660 (Walk 19)

The Saloon saloonmn.com, 830 Hennepin Ave., Minneapolis, 612-288-0459 (Walk 10)

St. Anthony Main Theatre stanthonymaintheatre.com, 115 Main St. S.E., Minneapolis, 612-331-4723 (Walk 15)

State Theatre hennepintheatretrust.org/our-theatres/state-theatre, 805 Hennepin Ave., Minneapolis, 612-339-7007 (Walk 10)

Stub and Herb's Bar and Restaurant stubandherbsbar.com, 227 Oak St. S.E., Minneapolis, 612-379-1880 (Walk 18)

Tom Reid's Hockey City Pub tomreidshockeycitypub.com, 258 7th St. W., St. Paul, 651-292-9916 (Walk 30)

Target Field minnesota.twins.mlb.com/min/ballpark, 1 Twins Way, Minneapolis, 612-338-9467 (Walk 13)

Triple Rock Social Club triplerocksocialclub.com, 629 Cedar Ave. S., Minneapolis, 612-333-7399 (Walk 8)

22nd Avenue Station Bar 2121 University Ave. N.E., Minneapolis, 612-789-6793 (Walk 19)

Uptown Theatre landmarktheatres.com/market/minneapolis/uptowntheatre.htm, 2906 Hennepin Ave., Minneapolis, 612-825-6006 (Walk 1)

The Varsity Theater & Café des Artistes varsitytheater.org/cafe, 1308 4th St. S.E., Minneapolis, 612-604-0222 (Walk 17)

Williams Arena umn.edu/twincities, 1925 University Ave. S.E., Minneapolis, 612-624-3514 (Walk 18)

Woman's Club of Minneapolis womansclub.org, 410 Oak Grove St., Minneapolis, 612-870-8001 (Walk 7)

Xcel Energy Center xcelenergycenter.com, 175 Kellogg Blvd. W., St. Paul, 651-265-4800 (Walk 30)

MUSEUMS & GALLERIES

American Swedish Institute/Fika asimn.org, 2600 Park Ave. S., Minneapolis, 612-871-4907 (Walk 6)

Bell Museum of Natural History bellmuseum.org, 10 Church St. S.E., Minneapolis, 612-624-7083 (Walk 18)

Como-Harriet Streetcar Line trolleyride.org, 2330 42nd St. W., Minneapolis, 651-228-0263 (Walk 3)

Frank Stone Gallery frankstonegallery.com, 1224 2nd St. N.E., Minneapolis, 612-617-9965 (Walk 19)

Grain Belt Bottling House and Warehouse artspace.org/our-places/grain-belt-studios, 77 and 79 13th Ave. N.E., Minneapolis, 612-465-0233 (Walk 19)

Hennepin History Museum hennepinhistory.org, 2303 3rd Ave. S., Minneapolis, 612-870-1329 (Walk 5)

Historic Streetcar Station tinyurl.com/historicstreetcar, 1224 Lexington Pkwy. N., St. Paul, 651-632-5111 (Walk 29)

Landmark Center landmarkcenter.org, 75 5th St. W., St. Paul, 651-292-3225 (Walk 31)

Mill City Museum millcitymuseum.org, 704 2nd St. S., Minneapolis, 612-341-7555 (Walks 12 & 15)

Minneapolis Institute of Arts artsmia.org, 2400 3rd Ave. S., Minneapolis, 612-870-3132 (Walk 15)

Minnehaha/Princess Depot mtmuseum.org/mhdepot.shtml, 4801 Minnehaha Ave. S., Minneapolis, 612-230-6400 (Walk 23)

Minnesota Children's Museum mcm.org, 10 7th St. W., St. Paul, 651-225-6000 (Walk 31)

Minnesota History Center mnhs.org, 345 Kellogg Blvd. W., St. Paul, 651-259-3900 (Walk 28)

Rogue Buddha Gallery roguebuddha.com, 357 13th Ave. N.E., Minneapolis, 612-331-3889 (Walk 19)

Science Museum of Minnesota smm.org, 120 Kellogg Blvd., St. Paul, 651-221-9444 (Walk 30)

Walker Art Center walkerart.org, 1750 Hennepin Ave., Minneapolis, 612-375-7622 (Walk 7)

Weisman Art Museum weisman.umn.edu, 333 River Rd. E., Minneapolis, 612-625-9494 (Walk 18)

Wells Fargo History Museum wellsfargohistory.com, 90 7th St. S., Wells Fargo Building, Minneapolis, 612-667-4210 (Walk 9)

EDUCATIONAL & CULTURAL CENTERS

Alliance Française afmsp.org, 113 1st St. N., Minneapolis, 612-332-0436 (Walk 14)

The Bakken: A Library and Museum of Electricity in Life thebakken.org, 3537 Zenith Ave. S., Minneapolis, 612-926-3878 (Walk 2)

Children's Theatre Company childrenstheatre.org, 2400 3rd Ave. S., Minneapolis, 612-874-0400 (Walk 5)

Cowles Center for Dance and the Performing Arts thecowlescenter.org, 528 Hennepin Ave., Minneapolis, 612-206-3636 (Walk 10)

Guthrie Theater guthrietheater.org, 818 2nd St. S., Minneapolis, 612-377-2224 (Walks 12 & 15)

In the Heart of the Beast Puppet and Mask Theatre hobt.org, 1500 Lake St. E., Minneapolis, 612-721-2535 (Walk 21)

James J. Hill Reference Library jjhill.org, 80 4th St. W., St. Paul, 651-265-5500 (Walk 31)

Macalester College macalester.edu, 1600 Grand Ave., St. Paul, 651-696-6000 (Walk 25)

MacPhail Center for Music macphail.org, 501 2nd St. S., Minneapolis, 612-321-0100 (Walk 12)

Minneapolis College of Art and Design mcad.edu, 2501 Stevens Ave., Minneapolis, 612-874-3700 (Walk 5)

Minnesota Vietnam Veterans Memorial mvvm.org, 20 12th St. W., St. Paul, 651-777-0686 (Walk 28)

Open Book openbookmn.org, 1011 Washington Ave. S., Ste. 100, Minneapolis, 612-215-2520 (Walk 12)

Orchestra Hall minnesotaorchestra.org, 1111 Nicollet Ave., Minneapolis, 612-371-5600 (Walk 11)

Ordway Center for the Performing Arts ordway.org, 345 Washington St., St. Paul, 651-282-3000 (Walk 31)

Pierre Bottineau Community Library hclib.org, 1224 2nd St. N.E., Minneapolis, 612-630-6890 (Walk 19)

Southeast Community Library tinyurl.com/secommlibrary, 1222 4th St. S.E., Minneapolis, 612-543-6725 (Walk 17)

St. Mary's University smumn.edu, 2500 Park Ave., Minneapolis, 612-728-5100 (Walk 6)

St. Paul Central Public Library tinyurl.com/stpaulcentrallibrary, 90 4th St. W., St. Paul, 651-266-7000 (Walk 31)

University of Minnesota umn.edu/twincities, 321 19th Ave. S., Minneapolis, 612-625-2008 (Walks 8 & 18)

William Mitchell College of Law wmitchell.edu, 875 Summit Ave., St. Paul, 651-227-9171(Walk 26)

HISTORIC HOUSES & BUILDINGS

Alexander Ramsey House mnhs.org/places/sites/arh, 265 Exchange St. S., St. Paul, 651-296-8760 (Walk 30)

American Swedish Institute/Fika asimn.org, 2600 Park Ave. S., Minneapolis, 612-871-4907 (Walk 6)

Ard Godfrey House tinyurl.com/ardgodfrey, 50 University Ave. N.E., Minneapolis, 612-870-8001 (Walk 16)

Basilica of Saint Mary mary.org, 88 17th St. N., Minneapolis, 612-333-1381 (Walk 7)

Cafesjian's Carousel ourfaircarousel.org, 1245 Midway Pkwy., St. Paul, 651-489-4628 (Walk 29)

Cathedral of Saint Paul cathedralsaintpaul.org, 239 Selby Ave., St. Paul, 651-228-1766 (Walk 26)

Church of the Assumption assumptionsp.org, 51 7th St. W., St. Paul, 651-224-7536 (Walk 31)

Church of the Holy Cross ourholycross.org, 1621 University Ave. N.E., Minneapolis, 612-789-7238 (Walk 19)

Como-Harriet Streetcar Line trolleyride.org, 2330 42nd St. W., Minneapolis, 651-228-0263 (Walk 3)

First Baptist Church fbcminneapolis.org, 1021 Hennepin Ave., Minneapolis, 612-332-3651 (Walk 10)

Hennepin Avenue United Methodist Church hennepinchurch.org, 511 Groveland Ave., Minneapolis, 612-871-5303 (Walk 7)

Holy Family Maronite Church holyfamilymaronitechurch.org, 203 Robie St. E., St. Paul, 651-291-1116 (Walk 32)

James J. Hill House mnhs.org/places/sites/jjhh, 240 Summit Ave., St. Paul, 651-297-2555 (Walk 26)

John Harrington Stevens House johnhstevenshouse.org, 4901 Minnehaha Ave. S., Minneapolis, 612-722-2220 (Walk 23)

Longfellow House tinyurl.com/houselongfellow, 4800 Minnehaha Ave. S., Minneapolis, 612-370-4969 (Walk 23)

Minnehaha/Princess Depot mtmuseum.org/mhdepot.shtml, 4801 Minnehaha Ave. S., Minneapolis, 612-230-6400 (Walk 23)

Minnesota State Capitol mnhs.org/places/sites/msc, 75 Dr. Rev. Martin Luther King Jr. Blvd., St. Paul, 651-296-2881 (Walk 28)

Our Lady of Lourdes Catholic Church ourladyoflourdesmn.com, 1 Lourdes Pl., Minneapolis, 612-379-2259 (Walk 16)

Plymouth Congregational Church plymouth.org, 1900 Nicollet Ave., Minneapolis, 612-871-7400 (Walk 4)

Saint Thomas More Catholic Church morecommunity.org, 1093 Summit Ave., St. Paul, 651-227-7669 (Walk 26)

S. S. Cyril & Methodius Catholic Church home.catholicweb.com/stcyril, 1315 2nd St. N.E., Minneapolis, 612-379-9736 (Walk 19)

St. Mark's Episcopal Cathedral ourcathedral.org, 519 Oak Grove St., Minneapolis, 612-870-7800 (Walk 7)

St. Mary's Greek Orthodox Church stmarysgoc.org, 3450 Irving Ave. S., Minneapolis, 612-825-2247 (Walk 2)

St. Paul's Evangelical Lutheran Church stpaulsevlutheran.org, 1901 Portland Ave. S., Minneapolis, 612-874-0133 (Walk 6)

Straitgate Church straitgate.org, 638 Franklin Ave. E., Minneapolis, 612-870-7472 (Walk 6)

Virginia Street Church virginiastreetchurch.org, 170 Virginia St., St. Paul, 651-224-4553 (Walk 26)

Westminster Presbyterian Church ewestminster.org, 1200 Marquette Ave., Minneapolis, 612-332-3421 (Walk 11)

Woman's Club of Minneapolis womansclub.org, 410 Oak Grove St., Minneapolis, 612-870-8001 (Walk 7)

SHOPPING

Aveda Day Spa Institute avedainstitutemn.com, 400 Central Ave. S.E., Minneapolis, 612-331-1400 (Walk 16)

Barnes & Noble bn.com, 801 Nicollet Mall, Minneapolis, 612-371-4443 (Walk 11)

Big Brain Comics bigbraincomics.com, 1027 Washington Ave. S., Minneapolis, 612-338-4390 (Walk 12)

Candy Alley candyalley.com, 4817 Chicago Ave. S., Minneapolis, 612-354-3881 (Walk 22)

Candyland candylandstore.com, 435 Wabasha St. N., St. Paul, 651-292-1191 (Walk 31)

City Center tinyurl.com/mncitycenter, 33 6th St. S., Minneapolis (Walk 9)

Common Good Books commongoodbooks.com, 38 Snelling Ave. S., St. Paul, 651-225-8989 (Walk 25)

Dahl Violin Shop 89 10th St. S., Ste. 205, Minneapolis, 612-339-4800 (Walk 11)

Dog Days dogdaysinc.com, 1752 Grand Ave., St. Paul, 651-642-9663 (Walk 25)

Dome Souvenirs Plus domeplus.com, 910 3rd St. S., Minneapolis, 612-375-9707 (Walk 12)

Dr. Chocolate's Chocolate Chateau drchocolate.com, 579 Selby Ave., St. Paul, 651-379-3676 (Walk 26)

Galtier Plaza galtierplaza.com, 380 Jackson St., St. Paul (Walk 31)

Gardner Hardware Co. gardnerhardwareco.com, 515 Washington Ave. N., Minneapolis, 612-333-3393 (Walk 13)

Gaviidae Common gaviidaecommon.com, 651 Nicollet Mall, Minneapolis, 612-372-1230 (Walks 9 & 11)

Half Price Books hpb.com, 2041 Ford Pkwy., St. Paul, 651-699-1391 (Walk 24)

Haskell's haskells.com, 81 9th St. S., Minneapolis, 800-486-2434 (Walk 11)

Highland Village Center tinyurl.com/highlandctr, 2024 Ford Pkwy., St. Paul (Walk 24)

Hmong Village 1001 Johnson Pkwy., St. Paul, 651-777-7886 (Walk 35)

IDS Center ids-center.com, 80 8th St. S., Minneapolis (Walks 9 & 11)

Ingebretsen's Scandinavian Gifts ingebretsens.com, 1601 Lake St. E., Minneapolis, 612-729-9333 (Walk 21)

Just Truffles justtruffles.com, 1363 Grand Ave., St. Paul, 651-690-0075 (Walk 25)

Kramarczuk's kramarczuk.com, 215 Hennepin Ave. E., Minneapolis, 612-379-3018 (Walk 16)

Love From Minnesota lovefrommn.com, 80 8th St. S., #178, IDS Center, Minneapolis, 612-333-2371 (Walk 9)

Mayday Books maydaybookstore.org, 301 Cedar Ave. S., Minneapolis, 612-333-4719 (Walk 8)

Melrose Antiques etsy.com/shop/melroseantiques, 13 5th St. N.E., Minneapolis, 612-362-8480 (Walk 16)

Mercado Central mercadocentral.net, 1515 Lake St. E., Minneapolis, 612-728-5401 (Walk 21)

Midtown Global Market midtownglobalmarket.org, 2929 Chicago Ave. S., Minneapolis, 612-872-4041 (Walk 21)

Midwest Mountaineering midwestmtn.com, 309 Cedar Ave. S., Minneapolis, 612-339-3433 (Walk 8)

Mill City Farmers Market millcityfarmersmarket.org, 704 2nd St. S., Minneapolis, 612-341-7580 (Walk 15)

Mississippi Market msmarket.coop, 622 Selby Ave., St. Paul, 651-310-9499 (Walk 26)

Red Balloon Bookshop redballoonbookshop.com, 891 Grand Ave., St. Paul, 651-224-8320 (Walk 25)

Seafood Market seafoodmarketmn.com, 628 Central Ave. S.E., Minneapolis, 612-379-6387 (Walk 16)

Sex World/Sinners shopsexworld.com, 241 2nd Ave. N., Minneapolis, 612-672-0556 (Walk 13)

Shop in the City 4737 Chicago Ave. S., Minneapolis, 612-825-2808 (Walk 22)

Stadium Village stadiumvillage.com, University Ave. S.E. and Huron Blvd. S.E., Minneapolis (Walk 18)

Tibet Store tibetstorempls.com, 2835 Hennepin Ave., Minneapolis, 612-872-8800 (Walk 1)

Uncle Hugo's/Uncle Edgar's unclehugo.com, 2864 Chicago Ave. S., Minneapolis, 612-824-6347/612-824-9984 (Walk 21)

Victoria Crossing 867 Grand Ave., St. Paul (Walk 25)

ParKS & GarDeNS

Beard's Plaisance Park tinyurl.com/beardsplaisance, 45th St. W. and Upton Ave. S., Minneapolis, 612-230-6400 (Walk 3)

Bohemian Flats Park tinyurl.com/bohemianflats, 2200 W. River Pkwy., Minneapolis, 612-230-6400 (Walk 18)

Boom Island Park tinyurl.com/boomisland, 724 Sibley St. N.E., Minneapolis, 612-230-6400 (Walk 14)

Boyd Park tinyurl.com/boydpark, 335 Selby Ave., St. Paul, 651-632-5111 (Walk 26)

Bruce Vento Nature Sanctuary nps.gov/miss/planyourvisit/ventosanctuary.htm, 4th St. E. and Commercial St., St. Paul, 651-266-6400 (Walk 34)

Calhoun Square calhounsquare.com, 3001 Hennepin Ave. S., Minneapolis, 612-824-1240 (Walk 1)

Chute Square tinyurl.com/chutesquare, 28 University Ave. S.E., Minneapolis, 612-230-6400 (Walk 16)

Cochran Park tinyurl.com/cochranpark, 375 Summit Ave., St. Paul, 651-632-5111 (Walk 27)

Community Peace Gardens koreanservicemn.org/programs/prog_farm.php, 808 Cedar Ave. S., Minneapolis, 612-342-1344, ext. 5 (Walk 8)

Como Park Zoo and Conservatory comozooconservatory.org, 1360 Lexington Pkwy. N., St. Paul, 651-487-8200 (Walk 29)

Currie Park tinyurl.com/mncurriepark, 500 15th Ave. S., Minneapolis, 612-230-6400 (Walk 8)

Edgewater Park tinyurl.com/edgewaterparkmn, 2326 Marshall St. N.E., Minneapolis, 612-230-6400 (Walk 19)

Father Hennepin Bluffs Park/Stone Arch Bridge tinyurl.com/hennepinbluffs, 420 Main St. S.E., Minneapolis, 612-230-6400 (Walk 15)

First Bridge Park tinyurl.com/firstbridgepark, 1 W. River Pkwy., Minneapolis, 612-230-6400 (Walk 15)

Ford Dam/Upper Mississippi River Locks and Dams No. 1 mvp.usace.army.mil, 5000 Godfrey Pkwy., Minneapolis (Walks 23 & 24)

Franklin Steele Square tinyurl.com/steelesquare, 1600 Portland Ave. S., Minneapolis, 612-230-6400 (Walk 6)

Gold Medal Park nps.gov/miss/planyourvisit/goldmedal.htm, 2nd St. S. and 11th Ave. S., Minneapolis, 612-230-6400 (Walk 15)

Gluek Park tinyurl.com/gluek, 2000 Marshall St. N.E., Minneapolis, 612-230-6400 (Walk 19)

Hamm Park tinyurl.com/hammpark, 743 7th St. E., St. Paul, 651-632-5111 (Walk 33)

Hidden Falls Park tinyurl.com/hiddenfallsmn, 1313 Hidden Falls Dr., St. Paul, 651-632-5111 (Walk 24)

Indian Mounds Park tinyurl.com/indianmoundsmn, 10 Mounds Blvd., St. Paul., 651-632-5111 (Walk 34)

Irvine Park tinyurl.com/irvineparkmn, 251 Walnut St., St. Paul, 651-632-5111 (Walk 30)

Lake Calhoun North Beach tinyurl.com/calhounnorth, 2710 Lake St. W., Minneapolis, 612-230-6400 (Walk 2)

Lake Harriet Southeast Beach tinyurl.com/SEbeach, 4740 Lake Harriet Pkwy. E., Minneapolis, 612-230-6400 (Walk 3)

Lake Nokomis tinyurl.com/lakenokomis, 4955 W. Lake Nokomis Pkwy., Minneapolis, 612-370-4923 (Walk 22)

Linwood Community Recreation Center tinyurl.com/linwoodparkmn, 860 St. Clair Ave., St. Paul, 651-298-5660 (Walk 27)

Longfellow Gardens tinyurl.com/longfellowgardens, 3933 E. Minnehaha Pkwy., Minneapolis, 612-370-4969 (Walk 23)

Loring Park tinyurl.com/loringlake, 1382 Willow St., Minneapolis, 612-370-4929 (Walk 7)

Lyndale Park tinyurl.com/lyndalepark, 4124 Roseway Rd., Minneapolis, 612-230-6400 (Walk 3)

Mears Park tinyurl.com/mearspark, 221 5th St. E., St. Paul, 651-632-5111 (Walk 31)

Midtown Greenway midtowngreenway.org, Abbott Ave. S. to W. River Pkwy. along Lake St. E., Minneapolis, 612-879-0103 (Walk 21)

Mill Ruins Park tinyurl.com/millruins, 103 Portland Ave. S., Minneapolis, 612-230-6400 (Walk 15)

Minnehaha Park tinyurl.com/minnehahapark, 4801 Minnehaha Park Dr. S., Minneapolis, 612-230-6400 (Walk 23)

Mississippi National River and Recreation Area nps.gov/miss, 120 Kellogg Blvd. W., St. Paul, 651-292-0200 (Walk 30)

Nicollet Island Park tinyurl.com/nicollet, 724 Sibley St. N.E., Minneapolis, 612-230-6400 (Walks 14 & 15)

North Loop Dog Grounds doggrounds.org, 3rd St. N. and 8th Ave. N., Minneapolis (Walk 13)

Parque de Castillo tinyurl.com/parquedecastillo, 149 Cesar Chavez St., St. Paul, 651-632-5111 (Walk 32)

Peavey Park tinyurl.com/peaveypark, 730 22nd St. E., Minneapolis, 612-230-6400 (Walk 6)

Phalen Park tinyurl.com/phalenpark, 1600 Phalen Dr., St. Paul, 651-632-5111 (Walk 35)

Rice Park tinyurl.com/ricepark, 109 4th St. W., St. Paul, 651-266-6400 (Walk 31)

Sam Morgan Prairie summithillassociation.org, 860 St. Clair Ave., St. Paul, 651-222-1222 (Walk 27)

St. Anthony Park tinyurl.com/stanthonypark, Jefferson St. N.E. and Spring St. N.E., Minneapolis, 612-230-6400 (Walk 15)

Summit Park tinyurl.com/summitparkmn, 185 Summit Ave., St. Paul, 651-632-5111 (Walk 26)

Swede Hollow Park swedehollow.org or tinyurl.com/swedehollow, 615 7th St. E., St. Paul, 651-632-5111 (Walk 33)

32nd Street Beach tinyurl.com/32ndbeach, 3200 Calhoun Pkwy. E., Minneapolis, 612-230-6400 (Walk 2)

Thomas Beach tinyurl.com/thomasbeach, Thomas Ave. S. and Calhoun Pkwy. W., Minneapolis, 612-230-6400 (Walk 2)

Tower Hill Park and Water Tower pperr.org/history/thetower.html, 55 Malcolm Ave. S.E., Minneapolis (Walk 20)

Upper St. Anthony Falls Lock and Dam nps.gov/miss/planyourvisit/uppestan.htm, 1 Portland Ave. S., Minneapolis, 612-333-5336 (Walk 15)

Washburn Fair Oaks Park tinyurl.com/wfopark, 200 24th St. E., Minneapolis, 612-230-6400 (Walk 5)

Water Power Park tinyurl.com/waterpwrpark, 204 Main St. S.E., Minneapolis, 612-230-6400 (Walk 15)

MISCELLANEOUS

Como Golf Course and Cross Country Ski Area tinyurl.com/comogolf or tinyurl.com/comoski, 1431 Lexington Pkwy. N., St. Paul, 651-488-9673 (Walk 29)

Como Lakeside Pavilion tinyurl.com/comopavilion, 1360 Lexington Pkwy. N., St. Paul, 651-488-4920 (Walk 29)

Eco-Yard Midtown hennepin.us/ecoyardtours, 22801 21st Ave. S., Minneapolis, 612-348-3777 (Walk 21)

Freewheel Bike freewheelbike.com, 2834 10th Ave. S., Minneapolis, 612-238-4447 (Walk 21)

Lakewood Memorial Cemetery lakewoodcemetery.com, 3600 Hennepin Ave., Minneapolis, 612-822-2171 (Walks 2 & 3)

McNamara Alumni Center mac-events.org, 200 Oak St. S.E., Minneapolis, 612-624-9831 (Walk 18)

Minneapolis Pioneers and Soldiers Memorial Cemetery friendsofthecemetery.org, 2945 Cedar Ave. S., Minneapolis, 612-729-8484 (Walk 21)

Minneapolis Queen **and** *Paradise Lady* twincitiescruises.com, Plymouth Ave. and Boom Island Park, Minneapolis, 612-378-7966 (Walk 14)

Minnesota Governor's Residence admin.state.mn.us/govres, 1006 Summit Ave., St. Paul, 651-201-3464 (Walk 26)

Minnesota Wild Hockey Club wild.nhl.com, 317 Washington St., St. Paul, 651-602-6000 (Walk 30)

Minnesota Zen Meditation Center mnzencenter.org, 3343 Calhoun Pkwy. E., Minneapolis, 612-822-5313 (Walk 2)

Phalen Park Golf Course golfstpaul.org, 1615 Phalen Dr., St.Paul, 651-778-0413 (Walk 35)

One on One Bicycle Studio oneononebike.com, 117 Washington Ave. N., Minneapolis, 612-371-9565 (Walk 13)

Saint Sabrina's saintsabrinas.com, 2645 Hennepin Ave., Minneapolis, 612-874-7360 (Walk 1)

INDEX

about the authors

Holly Day's writing has appeared in more than 3,500 publications internationally, including *Computer Music Journal*, *ROCKRGRL*, *Music Alive!*, *Guitar One*, *Brutarian Magazine*, *Interface Technology*, and *Mixdown Magazine*. Over the past couple of decades, her writing has received an Isaac Asimov Award, a National Magazine Award, and two Midwest Writer's Grants. Her books include *The Insider's Guide to the Twin Cities* and *Music Theory for Dummies*.

Sherman Wick is a native of the Twin Cities. Since receiving a history degree at the University of Minnesota, he's worked as a freelance writer and photographer, focusing on music, film, and Minnesota's rich cultural and historical offerings.

Holly and Sherman started writing their first book together, *The Insider's Guide to the Twin Cities*, one week after marrying. They live near downtown Minneapolis with their two children, Wolfgang and Astrid.